FRCA Part 2
MCQ Practice Exams

Mary Forsling Bsc PhD
Reader in Reproductive Physiology
Department of Gynaecology
St Thomas's Campus, UMDS, London.

Lesley Bromley Bsc MBBS FFARCS
Senior Lecturer in Anaesthetics
University College & Middlesex Medical School, London.

find more MCQ's in

– Craft, Upton
Key Questions in Anaesthesia
ISBN 1-85996-220-3   WO 218C

– B. Kumar MCQ's in
Anaesthesia : Basic Sciences
ISBN 0-7506-1556-7   WO28 K

PasTest
Knutsford
Cheshire

£ 13.95

© 1990 and 1995 PasTest
Egerton Court, Parkgate Estate, Knutsford, Cheshire WA16 8DX

First published 1991
This new edition 1995

A catalogue record for this book is available from the British Library.

ISBN 0 906896 33 9

Text prepared by Turner Associates, Knutsford, Cheshire.
Printed by Antony Rowe Ltd.

CONTENTS

PREFACE

The preparation of this book came about as a direct consequence of the success of its companion volume for the Part 1 FCAnaesthetists, by Drs Aveling and Ingram. We can assume that those using this book have already met the examiners at least once over the green baize, have heard their number called and later indulged in the gin and tonic and the carefree feeling of an exam safely behind them.

The career structure of anaesthetics in Great Britain does not allow the go-ahead young anaesthetist very long to rest on his or her laurels between taking the Part 1 exam and addressing the Part 2. This exam is a beast of a different nature to the Part 1. The Part 1 is designed to test a very broad general knowledge of the whole range of subjects which make up the specialty of anaesthesia. By contrast, the Part 2 exam is designed to test a very detailed knowledge of the scientific base on which anaesthesia is founded, concentrating specifically on physiology and pharmacology, but including a knowledge of statistics, and physiological measurement. In principle however it is no different from the Part 1 in that given sufficient preparation of the required subjects, the candidate who is well organised and presents the material in a competent manner will pass.

The Part 2 exam takes the form of a multiple choice question paper of 80 questions, roughly half of them cover physiology and the remainder pharmacology. There is nearly always at least one statistics question. While the broad emphasis is on those aspects of the subjects particularly relevant to anaesthesia, questions on any aspect of physiology and pharmacology can be asked, and the candidate should bear this in mind when preparing for the exam. In the exam paper the questions are grouped, with physiology presented first, followed by pharmacology.

In preparing these multiple choice questions, we have received invaluable help from junior anaesthetists who have recently taken the exam and others still preparing for it, while working with us in the Bloomsbury District both at The Middlesex Hospital and at University College Hospital. We are grateful to them for their feedback and useful advice on the exam from the consumer point of view.

Preparing for this exam requires a good deal of textbook study to learn the necessary facts. There is however no substitute for teaching by an informed senior, either on a one to one basis or in small groups, in order to acquire a true understanding of the facts. The principle of the Viva Voce exam technique is that if you truly know and understand a subject you will be able to explain it clearly to others. In other words viva practice is essential.

The vivas are held a number of weeks after the multiple choice paper and it requires some strength of mind to continue to read and prepare between the two parts of the exam. The two vivas last for twenty minutes each and are conducted by two examiners, each one will ask questions for roughly half the time available, although this is not a strict rule. One viva is devoted to physiology, and one to pharmacology, although statistics questions may be asked in either. The depth of knowledge asked for may be considerable, especially in subjects with close relevance to anaesthesia, however some breadth is also required so it is important not to read too narrowly during your exam preparation.

Finally, a well presented answer will give the required impression, and keeping a cool head when faced with an unusually phrased question will improve your chances of a pass. Remember that those whose knowledge may be encyclopaedic, can still fail if they are unable to present clear simple answers to the examiners' questions. Only allow the conversation to progress to the esoteric details once a good basic knowledge has been established. Thus we emphasise again the importance of viva practice. Adequate preparation, both of the information and of organised presentation, will see the candidate through the Part 2 and on to the final hurdle of the Part 3.

INTRODUCTION

Multiple Choice Questions are the most consistent, reproducible and internally reliable method we have of testing re-call of factual knowledge. Yet there is evidence that they are able to test more than simple factual re-call; reasoning ability and an understanding of basic facts, principles and concepts can also be assessed. A good MCQ paper will discriminate accurately between candidates on the basis of their knowledge of the topics being tested. It must be emphasised that the most important function of an MCQ paper of the type used in the FCAnaesthetists Part 2, is to rank candidates accurately and fairly according to their performance in that paper. Accurate ranking is the key phrase; this means that all MCQ examinations of this type are, in a sense, competitive.

The format of the multiple choice questions in the Part 2 follows the same pattern as that encountered in the Part 1. Each question consists of a stem and five items each of which in conjunction with the stem is either a true or a false statement. Candidates have to state whether the items are true or false. They may choose not to answer.

Examination Technique
The safest way to pass the Part 2 is to know the answers to all of the questions, but it is equally important to be able to transfer this knowledge accurately onto the answer sheet. All too often candidates suffer through an inability to organise their time, through failure to read the instructions carefully or through failure to read and understand the questions. First of all you must allocate your time with care. There are 80 questions to complete in 2 ¾ hours; this means approximately 2 minutes per question or 10 questions in 20 minutes. Make sure that you are getting through the exam at least at this pace, or, if possible, a little quicker, thus allowing time at the end for revision and a re-think on some of the items that you have deferred.

You must read the question (both stem and items) carefully. You should be quite clear that you know what you are being asked to do. Once you know this you should indicate your responses by marking the paper boldly, correctly and clearly. Think very carefully before making a mark on the answer sheet and take great care not to mark the wrong boxes. Regard each item as being independent of every other item - each refers to a specific quantum of knowledge. The item (or the stem and the item taken together) make up a statement. You are required to indicate whether you regard this statement as 'True' or 'False' and you are also able to indicate 'Don't know'. Look only at a single statement when answering.

Re-read the stem each time in conjunction with each branch as a complete statement and take care not to let the answer to one branch influence your answer to the other branches. This is the best way to avoid errors involving double negatives, much beloved of the setters of multiple choice exams.

It is impossible to overemphasise the fact that you must read the question carefully, re-reading the stem with each branch. The examiners have chosen the wording of the questions with much thought and deliberation. However, remember that in a clinical science absolutes are exceedingly rare, therefore words such as 'commonly' and 'may' abound in MCQ papers. Do not be put off by this or feel that the examiners are trying to trick you. If a question seems unclear and you are confused and do not understand, an examiner is present in the exam hall and you may ask for clarification.

Marking your answer sheets
Candidates receive +1 mark for each correct answer -1 for each incorrect answer and 0 for 'Don't know'. Thus the maximum mark for each stem is +5 and the minimum is -5.

The raw score is calculated from the number of correct and incorrect responses. The percentage score is calculated from the raw score by multiplying by 100 and dividing by the maximum possible score, in this case 400. The questions are all carefully assessed for their accuracy and degree of discrimination and their performance in the exam is reviewed on each occasion they are used. In this manner it is hoped to produce unambiguous questions and it can therefore be assumed that the obvious answer is correct.

The instructions to candidates given with the question paper should be read carefully. The answer sheet will be read by an automatic document reader which transfers the information it reads to a computer, it must therefore be filled out in accordance with the instructions.

As you go through the questions, you can either mark your answers immediately on the answer sheet, or you can mark them in the question book first of all, transferring them to the answer sheets at the end. If you adopt the second approach, you must take great care not to run out of time, since you will not be allowed extra time to transfer marks to the answer sheet from the question book. The answer sheet must always be marked neatly and carefully according to the instructions given. Careless marking is probably one of the commonest causes of rejection of answer sheets by the document reader. For although the computer operator will do his best to interpret correctly the answer you intended, and will then correct the sheet accordingly, the procedure introduces a possible new source of error. You are, of course, at liberty to change your mind by erasing your original selection and selecting a new one. In this event, your erasure should be carefully, neatly, and completely carried out.

Try to leave time to go over your answers again before the end, in particular going back over any difficult questions that you wish to think about in more detail. At the same time, you can check that you have marked the answer sheet correctly. However, repeated review of your answers may in the end be counter-productive, since answers that you were originally confident were absolutely correct, often look rather less convincing at a second, third or fourth perusal. In this situation, first thoughts are usually best and too critical a revision might lead you into a state of confusion.

To guess or not to guess
Do not mark at random. Candidates are frequently uncertain whether or not to guess the answer. However, a clear distinction must be made between a genuine guess (i.e. tails for True, heads for False) and a process of reasoning by which you attempt to work out an answer that is not immediately apparent by using first principles and drawing on your knowledge and experience. Genuine guesses should not be made. You might be lucky, but if you are totally ignorant of the answer, there is an equal chance that you will be wrong and thus lose marks. This is not a chance that is worth taking, and you should not hesitate to indicate 'Don't know' by leaving a blank if this genuinely and honestly expresses your view.

Although you should not guess, you should not give in too easily. What you are doing is to increase as much as possible, the odds that the answer you are going to give is the correct one, even though you are not 100% certain that this is the case. Take time to think, therefore, drawing on first principles and reasoning power, and delving into your memory stores. Do not, however, spend an inordinate amount of time on a single item that is puzzling you. Leave it, and, if you have time, return to it. If you are 'fairly certain' that you know the right answer or have been able to work it out, it is reasonable to mark the answer sheet accordingly. There is a difference between being 'fairly certain' (odds better than 50:50 that you are right) and totally ignorant (where any response would be a guess). The phrase

'MCQ technique' is often mentioned, and is usually used to refer specifically to this question of 'guessing' and 'Don't know'. Careful thought and reasoning ability, as well as honesty, are all involved in so-called 'technique', but the best way to increase the odds that you know the right answers to the questions, is to have a sound basic knowledge of medicine and its specialties.

Trust the examiners
Do try to trust the Examiners. Accept each question at its face value, and do not look for hidden meanings, catches and ambiguities. Multiple Choice Questions are not designed to trick or confuse you, they are designed to test your knowledge of medicine. Don't look for problems that aren't there - the obvious meaning of a statement is the correct one and the one that you should read.

Candidates often try to calculate their score as they go through the paper; their theory is that if they reach a certain score they should then be safe in indicating 'Don't know' for any items that they have left blank without needing to take the trouble to think out answers. This approach is not to be recommended. No candidate can be certain what score he will need to achieve to obtain a pass in the examination, and everyone will over-estimate the score he thinks he has obtained by answering questions confidently. The best approach is to answer every question honestly and to make every possible effort to work out the answers to more difficult questions, leaving the 'Don't know' option to indicate exactly what it means. In other words, your aim should always be to obtain the highest possible score on the MCQ paper.

Plan of campaign
You may have devised your own 'plan of attack' for multiple choice exams over the years, however we offer the following plan. You should consider it carefully, if only for the purpose of deciding on your own approach before you enter the exam hall.

1. Read the instructions on the exam paper with care.

2. Fill in your name and candidate number on the answer sheet.

3. Go through the paper and for each question:
    a) Read the question carefully.
    b) Mark on your question paper the answers which you are sure of, for example marking F for false and T for true next to the appropriate statements.
    c) Having been through the paper once marking all the responses

you know to be correct, start again at the beginning and spend some time trying to work out by reasoning those you are not sure of.

d) Any question which you feel you cannot answer should be left severely alone. Do not be tempted to guess.

4. Do not try to calculate the score you think you have obtained and then leave the remainder as 'Don't know', as you will always over estimate your correct score!

5. Remember to allow half an hour for filling in the answer sheet. Mark the sheet as instructed, double checking to be sure that you are doing so correctly. Transcription errors can occur by getting out of phase between the number of the questions on the paper and the numbers on the answer sheet, it is therefore worth marking five questions at a time, and then check them before moving on to the next five.

6. Leave a little time to go over the paper again, checking your transcription. Do not spend too much time at this stage rethinking answers you were originally sure about, as you will only become confused. Do not alter the answers on the computer sheet if at all possible.

7. Finally check that you have put your name and number on the computer sheet before handing it in. If you feel you have done all the questions you can, leave the hall and retire to the local hostelry for a reviving beverage!

MULTIPLE CHOICE QUESTION PAPERS

How to use this book

This book consists of four specimen multiple choice papers in pharmacology and physiology based on questions used in the actual exam. We would suggest that you work through each of these sets of 80 questions as if they were the real examination. You should spend no longer than two and a quarter hours on each paper, this will allow you a further half an hour to fill in the answer paper. Try to reproduce exam conditions, sit in a quiet place, and do not use any books.

As you work through each question, mark your answer against the space by the A. .B. .C. .D. .E. . at the bottom, using T for true and F for false. When you have completed the paper you can then mark it by using the answers. If you wish, you can calculate your raw score and percentage in the manner previously described.

Do not worry too much about your score, but rather use your overall performance to identify areas of weakness in your knowledge which can then be improved by further revision.

PRACTICE EXAM 1

80 Questions: time allowed 2 ¾ hours. Indicate your answers by putting T (True) or F (False) in the spaces provided.

1. **Active transport is involved in moving the following out of the cells:**
    A HCl from parietal cells
    B hormones
    C sodium
    D water
    E magnesium

    Your answers: A.....B.....C.....D.....E.....

2. **The following haemoglobin forms are seen in patients with β thalassaemia or sickle cell disease:**
    A HbA
    B HbF
    C HbM
    D HbH
    E HbS

    Your answers: A.....B.....C.....D.....E.....

3. **The cardiac index is**
    A cardiac output x body weight
    B cardiac output x total peripheral resistance
    C left atrial pressure – left ventricular pressure
    D cardiac output divided by surface area
    E stroke volume x surface area

    Your answers: A.....B.....C.....D.....E.....

4. **At an altitude of 4,600 m (15,000 ft), compared with sea level**
    A the partial pressure of water vapour in the alveolar air is down
    B the alveolar PO_2 is down
    C the percentage of oxygen inspired is halved
    D the alveolar PCO_2 is raised
    E the arterial blood oxygen saturation is unaltered

    Your answers: A.....B.....C.....D.....E.....

3

5. **Acidosis in uraemia is due to**

    A a failure to secrete hydrogen ions into the urine
    B a failure to secrete bicarbonate into the urine
    C a failure to form ammonia in the kidney
    D shortage of filtered buffer
    E production of aceto-acetate

    Your answers: A. . . . .B. . . . .C. . . . .D. . . . .E. . . .

6. **Calcium absorption**

    A may directly involve parathyroid hormone
    B is facilitated by lactose
    C occurs largely in the jejunum
    D is related to phosphate levels in the gut
    E depends on active transport mechanisms

    Your answers: A. . . . .B. . . . .C. . . . .D. . . . .E. . . .

7. **Hyperventilation occurs in the third trimester of pregnancy in association with an increase in**

    A $PaCO_2$
    B residual volume
    C oxygen consumption
    D circulating progesterone concentrations
    E metabolic acidosis

    Your answers: A. . . . .B. . . . .C. . . . .D. . . . .E. . . .

8. **When the motor nerve to a skeletal muscle is stimulated**

    A adrenaline is released from the nerve ending and depolarises the muscle
    B calcium enters the muscle fibres from the extracellular spaces during the plateau phase of the action potential
    C there is shortening of the myosin filaments
    D the muscle shortens at a speed proportional to the load opposing shortening
    E heat is liberated due to the inefficiency of the contractile machinery

    Your answers: A. . . . .B. . . . .C. . . . .D. . . . .E. . . .

9. **The knee jerk reflex**

   A   needs an intact spinothalamic tract
   B   has a single synapse in its pathway
   C   depends on the Golgi tendon apparatus
   D   depends on the γ efferent fibres
   E   is exaggerated in tetraplegics

   Your answers: A.....B.....C.....D.....E.....

10. **Magnetic resonance imaging**

   A   utilizes a weak magnetic field in conjunction with ionising radiation
   B   has tissue differentiating properties equal to ultrasound
   C   produces cross-sectional images reflecting proton density
   D   has abdominal image quality unaffected by respiratory motion
   E   is contraindicated in pregnancy

   Your answers: A.....B.....C.....D.....E.....

11. **Plasma volume can be measured using**

   A   para-amino hippuric acid
   B   inulin
   C   radioactively labelled albumin
   D   Evan's blue
   E   creatinine

   Your answers: A.....B.....C.....D.....E.....

12. **The Valsalva manoeuvre is associated with**

   A   an increase in pressure in the trachea
   B   a fall in the blood pressure initially
   C   a marked increase in the heart rate
   D   increased left ventricular stroke volume
   E   a fall in the right ventricular stroke volume

   Your answers: A.....B.....C.....D.....E.....

13. **The carotid body**

   A   contains chemoreceptor cells
   B   responds to a fall in pH
   C   has less blood flow than brain per gram of tissue
   D   responds to a fall in the partial pressure of oxygen more than oxygen content
   E   responds to a fall in blood pressure through it

   Your answers: A.....B.....C.....D.....E.....

14. **The following are permeable to water:**

   A   collecting duct in the presence of vasopressin
   B   ascending vasa recta
   C   ascending loop of Henle
   D   descending loop of Henle
   E   proximal convoluted tube

   Your answers: A.....B.....C.....D.....E.....

15. **Jaundiced patients may need parenteral vitamin K**

   A   as bile pigments degrade vitamin K
   B   as lack of bile pigments prevents its absorption
   C   as clotting may be disturbed in jaundiced patients
   D   given with bile salts
   E   vitamin K antagonises bilirubin

   Your answers: A.....B.....C.....D.....E.....

16. **The anterior pituitary gland secretes**

   A   growth hormone
   B   luteinising hormone
   C   oxytocin
   D   thyrotrophin releasing hormone
   E   glucagon

   Your answers: A.....B.....C.....D.....E.....

17. **Spermatozoa**

    A   require the presence of FSH for normal development
    B   fertilise the ovum within the uterus
    C   motile spermatozoa reach the uterine tubules faster than non-motile
    D   can release acrosin
    E   production is less at 38°C than at 36°C

    Your answers: A.....B.....C.....D.....E.....

18. **Stellate ganglion block causes**

    A   vasodilation in the ipsilateral arm
    B   pupil dilatation on the same side
    C   ptosis
    D   vasoconstriction of the contralateral leg
    E   parasthesia of the contralateral arm

    Your answers: A.....B.....C.....D.....E.....

19. **Fats are**

    A   components of cell membranes
    B   present in the diet as triglycerides
    C   absorbed by gut lymphatics
    D   found in the stools when bile secretion decreases
    E   required for prostaglandin synthesis

    Your answers: A.....B.....C.....D.....E.....

20. **A 20 kg child**

    A   has a reduced lung compliance compared to an adult
    B   has a blood volume nearer 3.5l than 1.5l
    C   has a mean arterial pressure of 80 mm Hg
    D   has a higher cardiac output on a weight basis than an adult
    E   has a higher GFR on a weight basis than an adult

    Your answers: A.....B.....C.....D.....E.....

21. **Alveolar-arterial oxygen difference is increased by**

    A high inspired oxygen
    B low inspired oxygen
    C breathing 0.003% carbon monoxide
    D a decrease in cardiac output
    E hypovolaemic shock

    Your answers: A. . . . .B. . . . .C. . . . .D. . . . .E. . . . .

22. **Surface tension is**

    A given by P x r/2 for a sphere
    B proportional to the square of the density
    C due to the cohesive forces between gas molecules
    D reduced by a rise in temperature
    E measured in dynes per square metre

    Your answers: A. . . . .B. . . . . .C. . . . .D. . . . .E. . . . .

23. **Inulin**

    A is freely filtered
    B is not reabsorbed
    C is secreted
    D is the same concentration in plasma as the filtered fraction
    E clearance is equal to that of urea when the urine flow rate is less
       than 1.5 ml/min

    Your answers: A. . . . .B. . . . . .C. . . . .D. . . . .E. . . . .

24. **Starvation in excess of 24 hours**

    A depletes glycogen stores
    B is associated with a markedly reduced blood glucose
    C is associated with a decreased lipolysis
    D is associated with a raised plasma tri-iodothyronine
    E is associated with an increase in urine acidity

    Your answers: A. . . . .B. . . . . .C. . . . .D. . . . .E. . . . .

25. Vasopressin secretion

A   is increased by alcohol
B   is increased by nicotine
C   is decreased by hypovolaemia
D   increases collecting duct permeability to water
E   is increased in response to an increase in plasma osmolality

Your answers: A. . . . .B. . . . . .C. . . . .D. . . . .E. . . . .

26. Gamma efferents

A   are co-activated with motor neurones
B   excite the uterus
C   cause mydriasis
D   are of limited usefulness in most voluntary actions
E   are involved in the control of breathing

Your answers: A. . . . .B. . . . . .C. . . . .D. . . . .E. . . . .

27. Experimentally during a tetanic contraction

A   each muscle fibre develops a greater tension than in a twitch
B   the tension is greater than in a twitch because more fibres are active
C   the muscle membrane is depolarised throughout
D   the intracellular calcium ion concentration reaches a higher level than in a twitch
E   the tension developed depends on the cytoplasmic calcium level achieved

Your answers: A. . . . .B. . . . . .C. . . . .D. . . . .E. . . . .

28. Cerebral blood flow

A   can be measured using the Fick principle
B   is normally 50 ml/100 g brain tissue/min
C   is greater through grey matter than white matter
D   is autoregulated by hypoxia stimulating the vasomotor centre
E   is increased by hypocapnia

Your answers: A. . . . .B. . . . . .C. . . . .D. . . . .E. . . . .

29. **In normal cerebrospinal fluid**

A PCO_2 is equal to arterial PCO_2
B   pH is equal to arterial pH
C   sodium is equal to plasma sodium
D   chloride is greater than plasma chloride
E   glucose is greater than the plasma glucose

Your answers: A.....B......C.....D.....E.....

30. **Cell membranes**

A   are composed of lipids
B   are permeable to water
C   are as permeable to glucose as urea
D   allow a passive chloride shift
E   pump Na^+ against a gradient

Your answers: A.....B......C.....D.....E.....

31. **In order to use Fowler's method to determine anatomical dead space the following are needed:**

A   expired PCO_2
B   inspired PCO_2
C   nitrogen analysis of expired air
D   inspired PO_2
E PaO_2

Your answers: A.....B......C.....D.....E.....

32. **In a patient lying on their side spontaneously breathing**

A   ventilation is greater on the dependent side
B   perfusion of the lungs is greater on the dependent side
C   the ventilation perfusion ratio is higher on the dependent side
D   there is increased shunting in the dependent lung with relatively lower PaO_2
E   there is an increased alveolar dead space in the lung that is dependent with increased $PaCO_2$

Your answers: A.....B......C.....D.....E.....

33. Muscle tone is

A   reduced if the ventral spinal root is sectioned
B   increased if the dorsal spinal root is sectioned
C   increased if the γ efferents are blocked
D   important for the maintenance of posture
E   due in part to the elasticity of the muscle

Your answers: A. . . . .B. . . . . .C. . . . .D. . . . .E. . . . .

34. Pulmonary blood flow

A   is distributed equally through the capillary beds
B   is decreased by sympathetic stimulation
C   is unchanged during exercise
D   is not influenced by changes of PO_2 in the alveoli
E   can be studied using intravenous radioactive xenon

Your answers: A. . . . .B. . . . . .C. . . . .D. . . . .E. . . . .

35. At 30 m of water for a diver

A   the lung is near the maximal expiratory position
B   the ambient pressure is 3 atmospheres
C   bubbles of nitrogen are formed in the tissues
D   the alveolar PO_2 is 28 mm Hg
E   there is an inflow of blood to thoracic organs

Your answers: A. . . . .B. . . . . .C. . . . .D. . . . .E. . . . .

36. The CO_2 response curve

A   is a plot of ventilation versus $PaCO_2$
B   has an intercept value just below the normal alveolar PCO_2
C   is shifted to the left with metabolic acidosis
D   has a decreasing slope with increasing hypoxia
E   is unaltered by respiratory depressant drugs

Your answers: A. . . . .B. . . . . .C. . . . .D. . . . .E. . . . .

37. The Frank-Starling mechanism (Starling's Law of the heart)

A   relates the force of contraction to the initial muscle fibre length
B   does not operate in the human heart
C   only operates in the denervated heart
D   can be masked by changes in contractility
E   serves to co-ordinate the output of the two ventricles as for example on assuming the upright posture

Your answers: A.....B......C.....D.....E.....

38. On changing from the supine to the erect posture

A   baroreceptor activity decreases
B   heart rate increases
C   left ventricular output increases
D   pressure in the leg vein increases
E   abdominal and limb flow falls

Your answers: A.....B......C.....D.....E.....

39. Regarding bone and calcium metabolism

A   chronic calcitonin generally causes hypocalcaemia in man
B   thickened osteoid seams are indicative of osteomalacia
C   elevated serum alkaline phosphatase is indicative of increased osteoclastic activity
D   vitamin D in high doses elevates plasma calcium even in the total absence of parathyroid glands
E   urinary hydroxyproline is an index of bone resorption

Your answers: A.....B......C.....D.....E.....

40. In patients with insufficient exocrine pancreatic secretion

A   fat digestion is normal provided bile is still produced
B   protein digestion is inefficient and loss of weight tends to occur
C   there is taken to be inadequate absorption of vitamins K and D
D   a bleeding tendency may be present
E   fasting blood sugar is elevated

Your answers: A.....B......C.....D.....E.....

41. The following antagonise insulin:

A   adrenaline
B   glucagon
C   growth hormone
D   propranolol
E   biguanides

Your answers: A.....B......C.....D.....E.....

42. The following are parasympathetic ganglia:

A   otic
B   sphenopalantine
C   stellate
D   ciliary
E   superior cervical

Your answers: A.....B......C.....D.....E.....

43. In summarising data

A   the mode is the value in the middle of a series of observations arranged in order of size
B   the median is the most commonly occurring value
C   the mean should generally be calculated
D   standard deviation is the measure of the difference of each observation from the mean
E   variance is the mean squared deviation

Your answers: A.....B......C.....D.....E.....

44. Heparin

A   is formed in the mast cells
B   reduces the conversion of fibrinogen to fibrin
C   is excreted by the kidneys unchanged
D   is absorbed from the gastro-intestinal tract
E   increases the prothrombin time

Your answers: A.....B......C.....D.....E.....

45. **Thyroxine is**

    A   bound to a protein in plasma
    B   a polypeptide
    C   is a factor contributing to skeletal growth
    D   antagonised by calcitonin
    E   is important in determining basal metabolic rate

    Your answers: A.....B......C.....D.....E.....

46. **Which of the following MAC values are correct? (in the absence of nitrous oxide):**

    A   halothane 0.76
    B   methoxyflurane 0.16
    C   ether 9.6
    D   cyclopropane 9.0
    E   enflurane 1.0

    Your answers: A.....B......C.....D.....E.....

47. **Pancuronium**

    A   causes less hypotension than curare
    B   crosses the placenta in insignificant amounts
    C   increases the heart rate
    D   dilates the pupil
    E   is potentiated by streptomycin

    Your answers: A.....B......C.....D.....E.....

48. **Sodium nitroprusside cyanide toxicity**

    A   is due to free cyanide ions
    B   is due to thiocyanate
    C   is worse in patients with vitamin B_{12} deficiency
    D   is worse in liver function impairment
    E   may result in worsening of symptoms in hypothyroid patients

    Your answers: A.....B......C.....D.....E.....

49. **Methaemoglobinaemia can result from the administration of**

    A   sodium nitrate
    B   methylene blue
    C   procaine
    D   prilocaine
    E   cinchocaine

Your answers: A.....B......C.....D.....E.....

50. **Hyperbaric oxygen can cause**

    A   painful joints
    B   pulmonary oedema
    C   acute tubular necrosis
    D   convulsions
    E   bradycardia

Your answers: A.....B......C.....D.....E.....

51. **The following agents are thought to lower blood pressure by acting centrally at or near the vasomotor centre:**

    A   hexamethonium
    B   propranolol
    C   amyl nitrate
    D   clonidine
    E   tubocurarine

Your answers: A.....B......C.....D.....E.....

52. **The following are recognised side effects of the named drugs:**

    A   amiloride – hypokalaemia
    B   morphine – diarrhoea
    C   phenytoin – megaloblastic anaemia
    D   phenacetin – renal papillary necrosis
    E   isoniazid – peripheral neuropathy

Your answers: A.....B......C.....D.....E.....

53. Labetalol

A   is a β receptor agonist
B   is an α_2 receptor antagonist
C   antagonises angiotensin
D   its β effects are longer lasting than its α effects
E   prevents release of noradrenaline from adrenergic nerve
    terminals

Your answers: A.....B......C.....D.....E.....

54. pH changes the structure of

A   atracurium
B   suxamethonium
C   gallamine
D   midazolam
E   diazepam

Your answers: A.....B......C.....D.....E.....

55. Warfarin levels are increased by

A   aspirin
B   cimetidine
C   phenylbutazone
D   rifampicin
E   griseofulvin

Your answers: A.....B......C.....D.....E.....

56. Prilocaine

A   is more effective topically than lignocaine
B   is less stable in solution than lignocaine
C   has a shorter duration of action than lignocaine
D   causes methaemoglobinaemia
E   is metabolised in the kidney

Your answers: A.....B......C.....D.....E.....

57. **The following drugs relax the pregnant uterus:**

A   salbutamol
B   adrenaline
C   noradrenaline
D   acetyl choline
E   dopamine

Your answers: A.....B......C.....D.....E.....

58. **Practolol**

A   cannot cause bronchoconstriction
B   increases exercise tolerance in angina pectoris
C   can cause keratitis
D   can cause sclerosing peritonitis
E   is a β adrenergic blocker

Your answers: A.....B......C.....D.....E.....

59. **Which of the following produce marked systemic analgesia:**

A   promethazine
B   fentanyl
C   pentazocine
D   thiopentone
E   chlorpromazine

Your answers: A.....B......C.....D.....E.....

60. **Atropine**

A   increases gut motility
B   is a mixture of D and L isomers
C   is equipotent with hyoscine
D   can cause bradycardia
E   crosses the blood brain barrier

Your answers: A.....B......C.....D.....E.....

61. **Dopamine receptor antagonists**

   A   increase heart rate
   B   are anti emetics
   C   cause hypertension
   D   cause extra-pyramidal side effects
   E   increase lower oesophageal sphincter tone

   Your answers: A.....B......C.....D.....E.....

62. **The following reduce gastric acid secretion:**

   A   ranitidine
   B   gastrin
   C   histamine
   D   adrenaline
   E   glycopyrrolate

   Your answers: A.....B......C.....D.....E.....

63. **Precursors of adrenaline include**

   A   noradrenaline
   B   metanephrine
   C   L-Dopa
   D   acetylcholine
   E   alanine

   Your answers: A.....B......C.....D.....E.....

64. **The action of curare is influenced by**

   A   a change of temperature
   B   a reduction in serum potassium
   C   aminoglycoside therapy
   D   ether
   E   pyridostigmine

   Your answers: A.....B......C.....D.....E.....

65. **Nitrates cause**

A reduction in CVP
B reduction in cardiac output
C increased meningeal blood flow
D reduction in pulmonary artery pressure
E increase in left atrial pressure

Your answers: A.....B......C.....D.....E.....

66. **The following dilate the pupils:**

A physostigmine
B pilocarpine
C trimetaphan
D guanethidine
E atropine

Your answers: A.....B......C.....D.....E.....

67. **The following are used in the treatment of ventricular arrhythmias:**

A digoxin
B disopyramide
C mexiletine
D tocainide
E verapamil

Your answers: A.....B......C.....D.....E.....

68. **The following drugs affect Ca^{++} levels in excitable tissue:**

A dantrolene
B nifedipine
C hydralazine
D halothane
E digoxin

Your answers: A.....B......C.....D.....E.....

69. **The following produce analgesia by an action on opiate receptors in the spinal cord:**

   A   aspirin
   B   epidural fentanyl
   C   acupuncture
   D   epidural bupivicaine
   E   rubbing the injured part

   Your answers: A.....B......C.....D.....E.....

70. **Significant vasoconstriction occurs with**

   A   cocaine
   B   procaine
   C   lignocaine
   D   amethocaine
   E   prilocaine

   Your answers: A.....B......C.....D.....E.....

71. **The following are true of dextrans in current use:**

   A   they are used for their calorific value
   B   the length of time they stay in the circulation depends on their molecular weight
   C   they can cause urticaria
   D   they are polysaccharides
   E   they are used in the prophylaxis of thrombosis

   Your answers: A.....B......C.....D.....E.....

72. **Uterine tone is**

   A   decreased by halothane
   B   increased by ketamine
   C   increased by β_2 agonists
   D   unaffected by neuromuscular blocking agents
   E   decreased by alcohol

   Your answers: A.....B......C.....D.....E.....

73. **Thiopentone is**

    A   the salt of a weak acid, and alkaline in solution
    B   is metabolised by mixed function oxidases
    C   is converted to pentabarbitone and excreted in this form
    D   has analgesic properties
    E   is stable in solution

Your answers: A.....B......C.....D.....E.....

74. **The following increase the amount of vapour which passes from alveoli to capillary blood:**

    A   altitude
    B   solubility of the vapour
    C   increased ventilation
    D   increased cardiac output
    E   rising alveolar concentration

Your answers: A.....B......C.....D.....E.....

75. **Suxamethonium is potentiated by**

    A   ecothiopate
    B   gallamine
    C   pilocarpine eye drops
    D   propanidid
    E   monoamine oxidase

Your answers: A.....B......C.....D.....E.....

76. **Aminoglycoside antibiotics can cause**

    A   optic atrophy
    B   dizziness
    C   ototoxicity
    D   potentiation of depolarising neuromuscular blocking drugs
    E   nephrotoxicity

Your answers: A.....B......C.....D.....E.....

77. **Absorption of drugs given by mouth**

    A can occur from the oral mucosa
    B is not affected by food intake
    C may be delayed by traumatic shock
    D is quicker after administration of atropine like drugs
    E is more rapid from the stomach than the small intestine for
       acidic compounds

    Your answers: A.....B......C.....D.....E.....

78. **Theophylline**

    A is a positive inotrope
    B increases glomerular filtration rate
    C causes bronchodilation
    D inhibits phosphodiesterase
    E causes cerebral depression

    Your answers: A.....B......C.....D.....E.....

79. **The following are solubilised in Cremophor E L (poly o-methylated castor oil):**

    A ketamine
    B althesin
    C etomidate
    D propanidid
    E diazepam

    Your answers: A.....B......C.....D.....E.....

80. **The following drugs exert an effect at the chemo-receptor trigger zone:**

    A digoxin
    B droperidol
    C morphine
    D metoclopramide
    E thiethylperazine

    Your answers: A.....B......C.....D.....E.....

PRACTICE EXAM 2

80 Questions: time allowed 2 ¾ hours. Indicate your answers by putting T (True) or F (False) in the spaces provided.

1. **Blood volume is maintained during severe hypovolaemia by**
   - A reduced neurohypophysial activity
   - B aldosterone
   - C angiotensin
   - D increased capillary hydrostatic pressure
   - E increased sympathetic nervous activity

   Your answers: A.....B.....C.....D.....E.....

2. **Tetany is associated with**
   - A hyperventilation at rest
   - B pyloric stenosis
   - C malabsorption syndrome
   - D a pancreatic fistula
   - E gluten sensitivity

   Your answers: A.....B.....C.....D.....E.....

3. **The sodium pump of cell membranes**
   - A is a sodium-potassium activated adenosine triphosphatase
   - B is inhibited by ouabain
   - C contributes to the low intracellular chloride ion concentration
   - D is responsible for the active transport of sodium ions into the cell
   - E is responsible for the generation of action potentials in nerve cells

   Your answers: A.....B.....C.....D.....E.....

4. **Haemoglobin**
   - A is a mucopolysaccharide
   - B each molecule reacts with four molecules of oxygen
   - C each gram of fully saturated haemoglobin combines with 0.003 ml oxygen
   - D is catabolised in the reticulo-endothelial system
   - E is a buffer in the blood

   Your answers: A.....B.....C.....D.....E.....

23

5. **Low ionised calcium concentrations in the plasma**

   A may be associated with an increased heart rate
   B have an excitatory effect on nerve and muscle cells
   C can result from hypoventilation
   D stimulate the secretion of the parathyroid hormone
   E stimulate the secretion of calcitonin

   Your answers: A.....B.....C.....D.....E.....

6. **Cardiac muscle differs from skeletal muscle in that cardiac muscle**

   A has a longer refractory period
   B responds in an all or nothing manner
   C can metabolise lactic acid
   D can only contract isometrically
   E can obtain a large part of its energy needs by anaerobic processes

   Your answers: A.....B.....C.....D.....E.....

7. **When $PaO_2 = 60$ mm Hg, $PaCO_2 = 30$ mm Hg, Base excess - 1, pH = 7.45, the condition is**

   A lactic acidosis
   B hypoxaemic hypoxia
   C compensated metabolic acidosis
   D hyperventilation
   E pulmonary atelectasis

   Your answers: A.....B.....C.....D.....E.....

8. **The cerebrospinal fluid**

   A is a pathway for the removal of the products of cerebral metabolism
   B contains less protein than plasma
   C is normally pale yellow
   D has a normal cell count of 50–100/ml
   E pressure may be 10 mm Hg in the lumbar area

   Your answers: A.....B.....C.....D.....E.....

9. **In a normal resting person**

   A   ventilation is controlled by PaO_2
   B $PaCO_2$ is controlled by pulmonary blood flow
   C   voluntary hyperpnoea increases the partial pressure of oxygen in the alveolus
   D   reducing ventilation causes an increased alveolar CO_2
   E   alveolar PCO_2 is virtually the same as mixed venous PCO_2

   Your answers: A.....B.....C.....D.....E.....

10. **Cardiac output**

   A   is increased by values of up to 35 l/min during exercise
   B   is increased by increasing vagal tone
   C   is decreased by noradrenaline infusion
   D   is increased by adrenaline
   E   may be increased when contractility increases

   Your answers: A.....B.....C.....D.....E.....

11. **Renal blood flow**

   A   is autoregulated
   B   is greater in the renal cortex than in the medulla
   C   can be measured using the Fick principle
   D   is approximately 10% of the resting cardiac output
   E   is unaltered by haemorrhagic states

   Your answers: A.....B.....C.....D.....E.....

12. **Calcium absorption in the gastro-intestinal tract**

   A   increases during lactation
   B   requires phosphate
   C   is passive
   D   depends on calcitonin
   E   is increased by 1,25 dihydroxycholecalciferol

   Your answers: A.....B.....C.....D.....E.....

13. In experimental hepatectomy the following occur:

A   a reduced blood urea
B   a fall in blood amino acids
C   hypoglycaemia
D   increased coagulability of the blood
E   bilirubin accumulation in tissues and blood

Your answers: A. . . . .B. . . . .C. . . . .D. . . . .E. . . . .

14. The excretion of acid in the urine

A   is under the control of aldosterone
B   varies with the ammonium output
C   varies with plasma inorganic phosphate
D   is reduced by inhibitors of carbonic anhydrase
E   is reduced in chloride depletion

Your answers: A. . . . .B. . . . .C. . . . .D. . . . .E. . . . .

15. A decrease in the effective circulating blood volume results in increased

A   rate of vagal discharge from volume receptors
B   secretion of vasopressin
C   fractional reabsorption of sodium in the kidney
D   urine volume
E   aldosterone secretion

Your answers: A. . . . .B. . . . .C. . . . .D. . . . .E. . . . .

16. Maternal changes during pregnancy include

A   an increased blood volume
B   an increased packed cell volume
C   increased plasma iron
D   reduced packed cell volume in pre-eclampsia
E   reduced plasma albumin concentration

Your answers: A. . . . .B. . . . .C. . . . .D. . . . .E. . . . .

17. The time course of the twitch of the adductor pollicis muscle on stimulation of the ulnar nerve is slowed when the hand is cooled because of

A   a slowed conduction velocity in nerve and muscle
B   a slower rate of interaction between actin and myosin
C   a reduced rate of uptake of calcium by sarcoplasmic reticulum
D   a reduced blood supply
E   a reduced release of acetylcholine at the muscle end plate

Your answers: A.....B.....C.....D.....E.....

18. Lesions of the cauda equinae can cause

A   sensory loss in the legs
B   paraplegia
C   abnormalities of bladder function
D   pain
E   loss of anal reflexes

Your answers: A.....B.....C.....D.....E.....

19. Given the following measurements:

Tidal volume 500 ml, rate of breathing 15/min
Dead space 100 ml, cardiac output 7 l/min

Which of the following statements is correct:

A   the pulmonary ventilation is 7.5 l/min
B   the subject is probably under 8 years old
C   the alveolar ventilation is 6 l/min
D   the ventilation perfusion ratio is the pulmonary ventilation divided by the cardiac output
E   the ventilation perfusion ratio is 0.86

Your answers: A.....B.....C.....D.....E.....

20. Ultrafiltration is responsible for fluid movement that takes place in

A   concentration of the bile
B   salivation
C   glomerular filtration
D   sweating
E   interstitial fluid production

Your answers: A.....B.....C.....D.....E.....

21. In the normal ECG with a rate of 80

A   the P-R interval is 0.11 sec
B   the QRS duration is 0.12–0.16 sec
C   the interval between each QRS complex is 0.75 sec
D   the S-T interval is 0.32 sec
E   protodiastole occurs over the Q-T interval

Your answers: A.....B.....C.....D.....E.....

22. Recognised effects of hyperbaric oxygen include

A   an increase in the oxygen content of the blood
B   supersaturation of haemoglobin
C   a fall in cerebral blood flow
D   convulsions only when the pressure exceeds 10 atmospheres
E   a decrease in cardiac output

Your answers: A.....B.....C.....D.....E.....

23. Stimulation of different regions of the hypothalamus could cause effects on

A   eating
B   water balance
C   temperature regulation
D   sexual activity
E   blood pressure

Your answers: A.....B.....C.....D.....E.....

24. An investigation on a woman aged 40 years gave the following results: (normal values in brackets)

haemoglobin 110 g/l (120–170)
Red cell count 3.2 x 10^{12} (4.5–6.5)
MCV 110 x 10^{-15}l (75–95)

A   the overall picture is normal
B   the findings are typical of iron deficiency
C   the findings are typical of vitamin B_{12} deficiency
D   this blood would carry about 150 ml O_2/l blood
E   the findings are typical of someone living at high altitude

Your answers: A.....B.....C.....D.....E.....

25. **In fetal circulation**

   A   the foramen ovale closes at birth because of an increase in the right atrial pressure
   B   blood in the descending aorta is less oxygenated than in the arch
   C   53% of the cardiac output goes to the placenta
   D   the pulmonary blood pressure increases at birth
   E   closure of the ductus arteriosus may be dependent on prostaglandins

   Your answers: A.....B.....C.....D.....E.....

26. **Lung compliance measurement**

   A   is a static measurement
   B   can involve the use of a spirometer
   C   can be performed using an interrupted technique
   D   gives a value at mid-lung volume of approximately 0.2 l/cm H_2O
   E   involves measurement of intratracheal pressure

   Your answers: A.....B.....C.....D.....E.....

27. **Compared to the A-V oxygen difference of 46 ml/l for the whole body, the value is lower in**

   A   heart muscle
   B   kidneys
   C   brain
   D   skin
   E   skeletal muscle

   Your answers: A.....B.....C.....D.....E.....

28. **The resting potential across the nerve membrane**

   A   depends on the ratio of the concentration of potassium ions inside and outside the cell
   B   is positive inside with respect to the outside of the cell
   C   is of the order of 0.08 volt
   D   decreases in magnitude during prolonged anoxia
   E   is larger the larger the diameter of the fibre

   Your answers: A.....B.....C.....D.....E.....

29. Chemoreceptors

    A   centrally respond largely to changes in plasma PO_2
    B   in the periphery respond to changes in PO_2
    C   peripherally respond to a low blood flow through them
    D   centrally are located in the hypothalamus
    E   impulses from the periphery all travel in the vagus nerve

Your answers: A.....B.....C.....D.....E.....

30. When urine is produced hypotonic to plasma there is

    A   an elevated glomerular filtration rate
    B   an augmented release of vasopressin
    C   active reabsorption of sodium in the renal tubule
    D   a low permeability to water in the collecting duct of the renal papillae
    E   shunting of the renal blood flow from medulla to cortex

Your answers: A.....B.....C.....D.....E.....

31. A patient secreting an excess of thyroid hormone would be expected to have

    A   a positive nitrogen balance
    B   increased blood cholesterol
    C   diminished urinary excretion of nitrogen
    D   increased pulse pressure
    E   heat intolerance

Your answers: A.....B.....C.....D.....E.....

32. Among the signs attributable to cerebellar lesions may be

    A   the inability to stop the arm from moving after it reaches its target
    B   the inability to maintain balance
    C   the inability to keep the arm from moving spontaneously
    D   muscle weakness
    E   the inability to perform rapidly alternating hand movements

Your answers: A.....B.....C.....D.....E.....

33. **The onset of puberty**

    A   has not occurred earlier with the progress of time, as myth would have it
    B   is accompanied by an increased secretion of adrenal androgens
    C   is when ova start to form in the ovum
    D   is accompanied by a pulsatile release of GnRH (LHRH)
    E   may occur early in children with hypothalamic lesions

    Your answers: A.....B.....C.....D.....E.....

34. **Acute right ventricular failure is accompanied by**

    A   raised central venous pressure
    B   enlargement of the liver
    C   normal jugular venous pressure
    D   reduced systemic arterial pressure
    E   increased aldosterone production

    Your answers: A.....B.....C.....D.....E.....

35. **The rate of pulmonary airflow during normal quiet breathing is influenced by**

    A   histamine
    B   dynamic airway collapse
    C   alveolar pressure
    D   intrapleural pressure
    E   autonomic nerve activity

    Your answers: A.....B.....C.....D.....E.....

36. **Hyponatraemia**

    A   can be seen in Addison's disease
    B   may occur in oat cell carcinoma of the bronchus
    C   may be seen in patients treated with chlorpropamide
    D   is always accompanied by dilute urine
    E   can lead to convulsions

    Your answers: A.....B.....C.....D.....E.....

E

37. **Afferent fibres travelling in the vagus to the heart**

    A   arise in the hypothalamus
    B   act on the heart cells via muscarinic receptors
    C   have nicotinic receptors in the peripheral synapse
    D   increase potassium conductance in the cardiac pacemaker cells
    E   decrease conduction velocity in the A-V node

    Your answers: A.....B.....C.....D.....E.....

38. **A patient is noted to have a markedly reduced colloid oncotic pressure and sodium excretion. After intravenous infusion of concentrated albumin solution, the patient has a rapid weight loss. It would appear that prior to treatment the patient had**

    A   enhanced K^+ excretion
    B   oedema
    C   an elevated aldosterone secretion
    D   a low secretion of vasopressin
    E   an elevated urine volume

    Your answers: A.....B.....C.....D.....E.....

39. **Pulse pressure increases as a result of an increase in**

    A   stroke volume
    B   heart rate
    C   arterial resistance
    D   peripheral resistance
    E   vagal tone

    Your answers: A.....B.....C.....D.....E.....

40. **After instilling dilute acid into the duodenum one would observe**

    A   secretion of bile
    B   secretion of pancreatic juices
    C   secretion of gastric juice
    D   release of secretin
    E   increased gastric motility

    Your answers: A.....B.....C.....D.....E.....

41. Insulin

A increases the entry of glucose into muscle cells
B enhances protein catabolism
C is a polypeptide hormone
D is secreted by the cells of the islets of the pancreas
E has a circulating half life of 12 h

Your answers: A.....B.....C.....D.....E.....

42. Of physiological solutions

A 0.9% saline is exactly isotonic with human plasma
B ammonium chloride may be used to treat metabolic acidosis
C 0.9% sodium chloride is a 0.15 M solution of NaCl
D ammonium chloride solution can precipitate a hepatic coma
E 0.9% sodium chloride can be used to maintain an isolated perfused heart in vitro

Your answers: A.....B.....C.....D.....E.....

43. Absorption of weak acids in the stomach

A is faster than that of weak bases
B is reduced in achlorhydria
C occurs at a rate directly proportional to the pH of gastric secretion
D involves diffusion of undissociated acid across the gastric mucosa
E occurs during gastrin, but not histamine induced gastric secretion

Your answers: A.....B.....C.....D.....E.....

44. Cortisol increases

A glycogenolysis in the liver
B gluconeogenesis by the liver
C free fatty acid metabolism
D the lymphocyte count in blood
E ACTH secretion via a feed back mechanism

Your answers: A.....B.....C.....D.....E.....

45. In statistical analysis

A the normal frequency curve is symmetrical around the midline
B the coefficient of variation is the standard deviation of the distribution expressed as a percentage of the mean of the distribution
C the standard error of mean is given by SD/n where n is the number of observations
D 75.73% of the population lies within one standard deviation
E 95.45% of the population lies within two standard deviations

Your answers: A.....B.....C.....D.....E.....

46. Beclomethasone

A can be given as an inhaler
B causes candidiasis
C raises plasma cortisol levels
D is a mineralocorticoid
E can produce adrenal suppression in children

Your answers: A.....B.....C.....D.....E.....

47. Atropine

A crosses into the central nervous system
B causes a bradycardia in small doses
C causes an increase in gastric emptying
D increases conduction through the AV node
E is a bronchodilator

Your answers: A.....B.....C.....D.....E.....

48. Morphine is metabolised by

A N-dealkylation
B conjugation and glucuronide formation
C hydrolysis
D oxidation
E N-deamination

Your answers: A.....B.....C.....D.....E.....

49. **When fentanyl is used during general anaesthesia the respiratory depressant effect**

    A   never outlasts anaesthesia
    B   is more readily reversed than analgesia, by naloxone
    C   may be diminished by pentazocine
    D   is due to reduced CO_2 production
    E   is augmented by opiate premedication

    Your answers: A.....B.....C.....D.....E.....

50. **Toxic impurities of nitrous oxide include**

    A   ammonia
    B   nitric oxide
    C   nitrogen dioxide
    D   thymol
    E   phosgene

    Your answers: A.....B.....C.....D.....E.....

51. **A competitive neuromuscular blocking drug would be**

    A   inhibited by hypokalaemia
    B   potentiated by neomycin
    C   unaffected by physostigmine
    D   potentiated by hypothermia below 30°C
    E   potentiated by magnesium excess

    Your answers: A.....B.....C.....D.....E.....

52. **β blockers**

    A   reduce pulse pressure
    B   reduce cardiac output
    C   are contraindicated in angina
    D   antagonise phenylepherine
    E   are contraindicated in diabetes mellitus

    Your answers: A.....B.....C.....D.....E.....

53. **Which of the following are true of thiopentone:**

A   a 2.5% solution has a pH of 6.8
B   more than 50% is protein bound
C   it is present at physiological pH in both ionised and unionised form
D   it is metabolised at less than 15% per hour
E   in small doses it is anti-analgesic

Your answers: A.....B.....C.....D.....E.....

54. **High molecular weight dextrans**

A   are polysaccharides
B   cause renal tubular necrosis
C   prevent thrombosis
D   are metabolised in the liver
E   have a half life of approximately 12 hours

Your answers: A.....B.....C.....D.....E.....

55. **Procaine has a short duration of action as a local anaesthetic because it**

A   is rapidly metabolised by plasma cholinesterase
B   causes local vasodilation
C   is more than 95% ionised at pH 7.4
D   has a low pKa
E   is rapidly excreted unchanged in the urine

Your answers: A.....B.....C.....D.....E.....

56. **Antibiotics**

A   penicillin is effective in meningococcal meningitis
B   penicillin resistant staphylococcus can be treated with flucloxacillin
C   aminoglycosides cause glomerular damage
D   septrin is bacteriocidal
E   chloramphenicol is useful in typhoid

Your answers: A.....B.....C.....D.....E.....

57. **The following are transmitter agents at autonomic ganglia:**

    A   acetylcholine
    B   adrenaline
    C   dopamine
    D   5 hydroxytryptamine
    E   noradrenaline

    Your answers: A.....B.....C.....D.....E.....

58. **The volume of secretions in the stomach is reduced by**

    A   antacids
    B   metoclopramide
    C   cimetidine
    D   atropine
    E   pyridostigmine

    Your answers: A.....B.....C.....D.....E.....

59. **Dopamine**

    A   is formed from L-dopa
    B   passes into the brain
    C   can cause arrhythmias
    D   causes hypertension
    E   causes nausea

    Your answers: A.....B.....C.....D.....E.....

60. **The following affect calcium flux:**

    A   digoxin
    B   hydralazine
    C   phentolamine
    D   diazoxide
    E   nifedipine

    Your answers: A.....B.....C.....D.....E.....

61. Mydriasis is caused by

A   ecothiopate
B   pilocarpine
C   homatropine
D   adrenaline
E   cyanide

Your answers: A . . . . . B . . . . . C . . . . . D . . . . . E . . . . .

62. The following can be used to treat digoxin induced dysrhythmias

A   propranolol
B   lignocaine
C   phenytoin
D   calcium chloride
E   potassium chloride

Your answers: A . . . . . B . . . . . C . . . . . D . . . . . E . . . . .

63. Competitive antagonism between two drugs occurs if

A   the agonist dose response curve is shifted to the right
B   the slope of the agonist log dose response curve is flattened
C   they act at different receptor sites
D   the maximal response to one is exactly halved by the other
E   they have equal and opposite effects

Your answers: A . . . . . B . . . . . C . . . . . D . . . . . E . . . . .

64. The anticoagulant action of warfarin

A   is exerted directly on the blood
B   is delayed in onset
C   can be reversed by vitamin K
D   is increased by phenylbutazone
E   is increased by concurrent administration of barbiturate

Your answers: A . . . . . B . . . . . C . . . . . D . . . . . E . . . . .

65. Frusemide

A decreases blood volume
B decreases blood sugar
C increases urate excretion
D decreases the hypertonicity of the renal medulla
E causes hypokalaemia

Your answers: A . . . . . B . . . . . C . . . . . D . . . . . E . . . . .

66. Heparin

A is a synthetic acid
B is found in mast cells
C is released during anaphylactic shock
D is an antiplasmin
E has a clearing action on lipaemic blood

Your answers: A . . . . . B . . . . . C . . . . . D . . . . . E . . . . .

67. The following relieve motion sickness:

A metoclopramide
B domperidone
C clyclizine
D imipramine
E hyoscine

Your answers: A . . . . . B . . . . . C . . . . . D . . . . . E . . . . .

68. A rise in blood sugar level can be due to

A glibenclamide
B diazoxide
C thiazides
D propranolol
E adrenaline

Your answers: A . . . . . B . . . . . C . . . . . D . . . . . E . . . . .

69. **The following are positive inotropic agents:**

    A   isoprenaline
    B   aminophylline
    C   merphentermine
    D   methoxamine
    E   labetalol

    Your answers: A.....B.....C.....D.....E.....

70. **The following drugs can adversely react with monoamine oxidase inhibitors:**

    A   pethidine
    B   amitriptyline
    C   ephedrine
    D   tubocurarine
    E   halothane

    Your answers: A.....B.....C.....D.....E.....

71. **Histamine can be released by**

    A   trimetaphan camsylate
    B   chlorpheniramine
    C   metoclopramide
    D   promethazine
    E   morphine

    Your answers: A.....B.....C.....D.....E.....

72. **Competitive neuromuscular block is potentiated by**

    A   lithium
    B   trimetaphan
    C   suxamethonium
    D   diazepam
    E   ether

    Your answers: A.....B.....C.....D.....E.....

73. **Cinchocaine**

    A   is a cinchona alkaloid
    B   is a potent local anaesthetic
    C   has an ester linkage and cannot be autoclaved
    D   has been widely used for spinal anaesthesia
    E   is used in a test for atypical pseudocholinesterase

    Your answers: A.....B.....C.....D.....E.....

74. **Opioid receptors**

    A   are found exclusively in the brain
    B   morphine acts principally at the mu receptors
    C   kappa receptor agonists are associated with dysphoria
    D   β endorphins are the naturally occurring agonists at the mu receptors
    E   naloxone is an antagonist at kappa receptors only

    Your answers: A.....B.....C.....D.....E.....

75. **The following are neurotransmitters in the central nervous system:**

    A   noradrenaline
    B   GABA
    C   glycine
    D   5-hydroxytryptamine
    E   acetylcholine

    Your answers: A.....B.....C.....D.....E.....

76. **Aspirin overdosage causes**

    A   thrombocytopenia
    B   coma
    C   metabolic acidosis
    D   jaundice
    E   pulmonary oedema

    Your answers: A.....B.....C.....D.....E.....

77. Drugs which undergo significant first pass metabolism include

A   morphine
B   buprenorphine
C   lignocaine
D   warfarin
E   aspirin

Your answers: A.....B.....C.....D.....E.....

78. Ketamine causes

A   bradycardia
B   postural hypotension
C   increased intracranial pressure
D   hallucinations
E   muscle rigidity

Your answers: A.....B.....C.....D.....E.....

79. The minimum alveolar concentration (MAC) of an anaesthetic agent is

A   increased in neonates
B   reduced in the elderly
C   reduced by fentanyl
D   affected by verapamil
E   reduced by nifedipine

Your answers: A.....B.....C.....D.....E.....

80. Atracurium

A   is metabolised by ester hydrolysis
B   metabolism is slowed by hypothermia
C   is broken down to laudanosine
D   in large doses is faster acting than suxamethonium
E   a decrease in pH will increase its shelf half life

Your answers: A.....B.....C.....D.....E.....

PRACTICE EXAM 3

80 Questions: time allowed 2¾ hours. Indicate your answers by putting T (True) or F (False) in the spaces provided.

1. **The P50 (PO_2 at which haemoglobin is half saturated with oxygen)**

   A   for normal arterial blood is 27 mm Hg
   B   is increased when blood pH falls
   C   is unaffected by the operation of the Bohr effect
   D   is increased by increased 2,3 diphosphoglycerate
   E   is increased by ascending to high altitudes

   Your answers: A.....B.....C.....D.....E.....

2. **For cardiac muscle**

   A   action potentials propagate from one muscle fibre to another
   B   the action potential lasts almost as long as the mechanical response
   C   normal heart beats are neurogenic in origin
   D   a fused tetanic response can be produced by repetitive stimulation
   E   spontaneous contraction occurs in the muscle due to the presence of pacemaker cells

   Your answers: A.....B.....C.....D.....E.....

3. **The following results: pH 7.43, $PaCO_2$ = 6.4 kPa, plasma bicarbonate 43 mmol/l could be caused by:**

   A   uncompensated alkalosis
   B   uncompensated metabolic acidosis
   C   compensated metabolic alkalosis
   D   compensated respiratory acidosis
   E   compensated respiratory alkalosis

   Your answers: A.....B.....C.....D.....E.....

4. **Vasodilatation in one arm is caused by**

   A   drinking milk at 50°C
   B   dipping the other arm in hot water
   C   standing up from a supine position
   D   a fall in PaO_2
   E   a rise in PCO_2

   Your answers: A.....B.....C.....D.....E.....

5. **Total gastrectomy could lead to**

   A   haemodilution after drinking water due to excessively rapid reabsorption
   B   malabsorption of protein due to lack of pepsin
   C   vitamin B_{12} malabsorption
   D   some impairment of carbohydrate absorption
   E   iron deficiency

   Your answers: A.....B.....C.....D.....E.....

6. **As compared with the initial conditions, following haemorrhage**

   A   tissue fluid formation increases
   B   heart rate increases
   C   cardiac output increases
   D   venous capacitance decreases
   E   renal blood flow decreases

   Your answers: A.....B.....C.....D.....E.....

7. **Functional residual capacity**

   A   equals the sum of the residual volume plus the inspiratory reserve volume
   B   is not influenced by posture
   C   is the volume at which some airways may close on expiration
   D   is a measure of the resting expiratory position
   E   measurement involves a helium dilution method

   Your answers: A.....B.....C.....D.....E.....

8. **Thermoregulation**

   A   involves hypothalamic receptors
   B   control occurs in the medulla
   C   involves fibres running in the lateral spinothalamic tract
   D   is important as a rise in temperature to 40°C results in marked apathy and impaired judgement
   E   may occur at the expense of fluid balance

   Your answers: A.....B.....C.....D.....E.....

9. **The major factor limiting expiratory flow rate during most of a maximal forced expiration is**

A   maximal velocity of contraction of intercostal muscles
B   turbulence of peripheral airways
C   turbulence of central airways
D   compression of the airways
E   contraction of the diaphragm

Your answers: A.....B.....C.....D.....E.....

10. **Compared to the fluid in the glomerular capsule, the filtrate in the juxtaglomerular nephron by the time it has reached the end of the proximal tubule may have**

A   a higher concentration of PAH
B   a higher concentration of inulin
C   a lower osmotic pressure
D   a lower urea concentration
E   a higher concentration of NH_4^+

Your answers: A.....B.....C.....D.....E.....

11. **It is possible to observe in patients with hypothyroidism**

A   hirsutism
B   a reduced sublingual temperature
C   moist hands
D   a tendency to fall asleep
E   a husky voice

Your answers: A.....B.....C.....D.....E.....

12. **Regarding the fetus**

A   IgG antibodies are transferred to it across the placenta, probably by pinocytosis
B   insulin in the blood is derived mainly from its own pancreas
C   fat is synthesised from glucose acetate and free fatty acids which have been actively transported across the placenta
D   most drugs will cross the placenta to some extent
E   fat soluble vitamins are readily transported across the placenta

Your answers: A.....B.....C.....D.....E.....

13. **Concerning the ear and hearing**

    A a greater displacement of the basilar membrane is perceived as a louder sound
    B there is a linear relationship between increases in sound pressure and the perceived increase in loudness
    C the oval window, but not the round window vibrates when sound is conducted by the ossicles
    D a loud sound will excite the parasympathetic nervous system
    E the auditory cortex is necessary for the discrimination of temporal patterns of sounds (tunes)

    Your answers: A.....B.....C.....D.....E.....

14. **Ascites may result from**

    A reduced central venous pressure
    B portal hypertension
    C reduced renal excretion of sodium ions
    D damage to liver parenchyma
    E hypoalbuminaemia

    Your answers: A.....B.....C.....D.....E.....

15. **The haemoglobin-oxygen dissociation curve moves to the right**

    A with a rise in temperature
    B with a rise in pH
    C in the pulmonary capillary
    D with carbon monoxide poisoning
    E with an increase in 2,3 diphosphoglycerate

    Your answers: A.....B.....C.....D.....E.....

16. **Reduced pulmonary vascular resistance may be produced by**

    A living at an altitude of 15,000 ft
    B inspiration to total lung capacity
    C moderate exercise
    D expiration to residual volume
    E right ventricular hypertrophy

    Your answers: A.....B.....C.....D.....E.....

17. **Oxygen consumption of cardiac muscle is increased by an increase in**

    A   activity of the parasympathetic nerves to the heart
    B   activity of the sympathetic nerves to the heart
    C   heart size
    D   heart rate by artificial pacemaker
    E   systemic arterial blood pressure

    Your answers: A.....B.....C.....D.....E.....

18. **Regarding respiration**

    A   the external intercostals and diaphragm are inspiratory
    B   transection of the spinal cord at C5 would prevent breathing
    C   forced expiration would be severely limited by a C8 transection
    D   the diaphragm is composed largely of smooth muscle
    E   section of the spinal cord at C1 would completely paralyse the respiratory muscles

    Your answers: A.....B.....C.....D.....E.....

19. **A decrease in the filtration fraction is produced by**

    A   decreased arterial plasma colloid oncotic pressure
    B   increased ureteral pressure
    C   increased efferent arteriolar resistance
    D   decreased filtration area
    E   decreased glomerular capillary pressure

    Your answers: A.....B.....C.....D.....E.....

20. **During absorption in the gut**

    A   all calcium is absorbed
    B   undigested protein is never absorbed
    C   fatty acids and triglycerides after entering the mucosal cell are resynthesised into triglycerides
    D   amino acids are nearly all absorbed actively
    E   most water reabsorption takes place in the colon

    Your answers: A.....B.....C.....D.....E.....

21. **In acute glaucoma**

    A   the iridocorneal angles becomes blocked
    B   blood flow through the retina is impaired
    C   intraocular pressure may be increased to a maximum of 25 mm Hg
    D   intraocular pressure may be reduced by the administration of atropine
    E   intraocular pressure increases on administration of carbonic anhydrase inhibitors

    Your answers: A.....B.....C.....D.....E.....

22. **Functions of pulmonary surfactant include a reduction of**

    A   lung compliance
    B   filtration forces from the capillary
    C   the surface tension of the lungs
    D   transpulmonary pressure
    E   alveolar radius

    Your answers: A.....B.....C.....D.....E.....

23. **Transferrin**

    A   is a protein iron complex in interstitial epithelial cells functioning as a store of iron
    B   transfers iron from gut to bone marrow
    C   transfers iron from gut lumen to marrow stores
    D   is a polypeptide
    E   in plasma is normally fully saturated with iron

    Your answers: A.....B.....C.....D.....E.....

24. **As a result of the pleural pressure gradient from the base to the apex of the lung**

    A   the pulmonary blood flow is unevenly distributed
    B   the apical alveoli are more inflated than those at the base
    C   the apical alveoli receive the largest portion of the tidal volume
    D   the basal airways close off first during expiration
    E   the ventilation perfusion ratio falls from base to apex

    Your answers: A.....B.....C.....D.....E.....

25. **Contrast media used for X-ray urography**

A give better contrast in a dehydrated subject
B are actively secreted in the distal tubule
C give better contrast in renal failure
D are not filtered in the kidney
E may contain iodine

Your answers: A.....B.....C.....D.....E.....

26. **The human myometrium in the proliferative phase is characterised by**

A reconstruction of cellular tissue and glands
B the glands becoming corkscrew-like and beginning to secrete
C firm tissue with little or no oedematous swelling
D great vascular development
E bleeding and shedding of superficial layers

Your answers: A.....B.....C.....D.....E.....

27. **The renal circulation**

A has a high blood flow relative to oxygen requirements
B is autoregulated
C requires a blood flow of 120 ml/min
D shows no alteration in flow on exercise
E receives increased flow on hypoxia

Your answers: A.....B.....C.....D.....E.....

28. **In tests of blood coagulation**

A the clotting time is 6–12 min in siliconised tubes
B the normal prothrombin clotting time (Quicks one stage test) is 11–16 sec
C the prothrombin time is normal in patients with haemophilia
D clot retraction takes palce within 24 hours in patients with haemophilia
E intrinsic thromoplastin formation is normal in thrombo-cytopenia

Your answers: A.....B.....C.....D.....E.....

29. Blood oxygen tension may be determined using

A   a Haldane apparatus
B   a Roughton Scholander apparatus
C   platinum electrodes
D O_2 light absorption using monochromatic red light of wavelength 630×10^{-9} m
E   a paramagnetic oxygen analyser

Your answers: A.....B.....C.....D.....E.....

30. Peristalsis is notable in the

A   oesophagus
B   proximal stomach
C   distal stomach
D   small intestine
E   colon

Your answers: A.....B.....C.....D.....E.....

31. It is possible to induce the appearance of an abnormal EEG by

A   having the patient close their eyes
B   tilting the patient to the supine position
C   asking the patient to perform arithmetic calculations
D   inducing alkalosis by forced hyperventilation
E   altering plasma vasopressin concentrations

Your answers: A.....B.....C.....D.....E.....

32. Voluntary hyperventilation continued for a period of 5 min results in

A   reduced availability of oxygen to the brain
B   decreased PO_2 of arterial blood
C   raised blood pH
D   raised PCO_2 of arterial blood
E   arterial hypertension

Your answers: A.....B.....C.....D.....E.....

33. Factors which increase the stiffness of arterial walls

A   decrease the velocity of the pulse wave
B   give a rapid and extensive rise in the amplitude of the pulse wave with a gradual diastolic decrease
C   lead to a rise in diastolic pressure
D   lead to an increase in peripheral resistance
E   lead to an increase in the systolic arterial pressure

Your answers: A.....B.....C.....D.....E.....

34. When the sole of the foot is stroked firmly

A   in a normal person the great toe shows plantar flexion
B   the opposite leg may extend in a patient with long standing spinal cord section
C   it may trigger widespread flexor reflexes
D   dorsiflexion of the great toe indicates a pyramidal tract lesion
E   the great toe tends to dorsiflex when the foot is affected by a lower motor lesion

Your answers: A.....B.....C.....D.....E.....

35. Retention of sodium is associated with

A   the first three days after a major surgical operation
B   a rise in the hydrostatic pressure in the capillaries
C   an increase in the percentage of body weight in the extracellular compartment
D   glucocorticoid administration
E   elevated vasopressin concentrations

Your answers: A.....B.....C.....D.....E.....

36. Over the respiratory cycle

A   the intrapleural pressure is -10 cm water at the end of expiration
B   resistance forces are zero at the end of inspiration
C   intrapleural pressure exceeds zero at the end of forced expiration
D   on inspiration the fall in intrapleural pressure is due to elastic recoil
E   alveolar pressure is elevated at the onset of respiration

Your answers: A.....B.....C.....D.....E.....

37. **A 40-year-old man at rest may have all his daily caloric needs met by (all figures in grams)**

	Fat	Carbohydrate	Protein
A	100	375	100
B	145	300	50
C	140	100	50
D	70	50	200
E	140	140	200

Your answers: A.....B.....C.....D.....E.....

38. **An anatomical shunt**

A   is the blood in the systemic arteries returning from the lung parenchyma and myocardium

B   can be distinguished from a physiological shunt by the use of 100% O_2

C   when given pure O_2 results in an increase in the oxygen content of the blood

D   when given pure O_2 the PaO_2 is raised to the normal value

E   is about 1–2% of the cardiac output

Your answers: A.....B.....C.....D.....E.....

39. **Loss of fluid from pulmonary capillaries**

A   does not occur in the healthy lung

B   increases if there is deficient surfactant

C   necessarily results in movement of fluid into the alveoli

D   is increased with increases in pulmonary blood flow

E   increases with increased pulmonary capillary pressure

Your answers: A.....B.....C.....D.....E.....

40. **Intracranial pressure**

A   rises in a Valsalva manoeuvre

B   rises when arterial CO_2 pressure falls below normal

C   when increased tends to produce cupping of the optic disc with the disc bulging backwards away from the vitreous humour

D   when increased may cause squinting and loss of the sensation of smell in children

E   when dangerously high, cerebrospinal fluid should be removed by lumbar puncture if depressed respiration is noted

Your answers: A.....B.....C.....D.....E.....

41. Aldosterone

    A   is a polypeptide
    B   is synthesised in the zona glomerulosa of the adrenal cortex
    C   acts on the epithelium of the proximal tubule
    D   increases urinary K^+
    E   increases urinary pH

Your answers: A.....B.....C.....D.....E.....

42. Comparing means should be performed using

    A   Student's t test for independent samples
    B   the Mann Whitney U-test
    C   the Wilcoxan matched pairs signed rank test
    D   the paired t test
    E   the method of least squares

Your answers: A.....B.....C.....D.....E.....

43. Local application of atropine to the eyes

    A   leads to dilation of the pupils
    B   causes difficulty in looking upwards
    C   results in impaired ability to focus on near objects
    D   results in a reduction of aqueous humour outflow
    E   should be avoided when glaucoma is suspected

Your answers: A.....B.....C.....D.....E.....

44. Precursors of adrenaline are

    A   tyrosine
    B   dopamine
    C   phenylalanine
    D   noradrenaline
    E   isoprenaline

Your answers: A.....B.....C.....D.....E.....

45. **In patients who have received high dose corticosteroid therapy**

A   ACTH administration during therapy prevents steroid withdrawal symptoms on its cessation

B   pituitary adrenocortical suppression is not usually observed if the dose of prednisolone is 7.5 mg

C   on its discontinuation pituitary ACTH secretion recovers before adrenocortical responsiveness to ACTH

D   alternate day drug therapy depends on differing duration of the actions of cortisol

E   alternate day steroid therapy is of no benefit in preventing adrenocortical suppression

Your answers: A.....B.....C.....D.....E.....

46. **Ethrane**

A   is a fluorinated hydrocarbon

B   has a boiling point close to halothane

C   potentiates curare

D   is metabolised to a small quantity of free fluoride ions

E   is more potent than halothane

Your answers: A.....B.....C.....D.....E.....

47. **Nifedipine causes**

A   tremor

B   increased cardiac output

C   vasodilation

D   it can be absorbed sublingually

E   decreased coronary vascular resistance

Your answers: A.....B.....C.....D.....E.....

48. **Topical application of anticholinesterase to the eye causes**

A   miosis

B   reduced tear formation

C   ciliary muscle spasm

D   conjunctival hyperaemia

E   loss of accommodation

Your answers: A.....B.....C.....D.....E.....

49. Dantrolene

  A has muscle relaxant properties
  B is useful in the treatment of malignant hyperpyrexia
  C inhibits myoneural blocking drugs
  D is an opiate antagonist
  E is an analeptic agent

Your answers: A.....B.....C.....D.....E.....

50. Glyceryl trinitrate (GTN) causes

  A meningeal venodilatation
  B fall in central venous pressure
  C fall in pulmonary artery pressure
  D venodilatation
  E coronary vasodilatation

Your answers: A.....B.....C.....D.....E.....

51. The following cause diarrhoea:

  A codeine
  B cimetidine
  C magnesium sulphate
  D phenytoin
  E dioctyl sodium sulphosuccinate

Your answers: A.....B.....C.....D.....E.....

52. Dopamine hydrochloride

  A is a negative inotropic agent
  B increases renal blood flow in low doses
  C has a stimulating effect on the central nervous system
  D is a beta blocker
  E is thought to act on dopaminergic receptors

Your answers: A.....B.....C.....D.....E.....

53. **The following are mechanisms by which transmitter action can be terminated at mammalian neuro-effector junctions:**

    A   neuronal re-uptake
    B   oxidation by diamine oxidase
    C   conjugation by choline acetyltransferase
    D   hydrolysis by butrylcholinesterase
    E   hydrolysis by acetylcholinesterase

    Your answers: A. . . . .B. . . . .C. . . .D. . . . .E. . . . .

54. **The following antibiotics have clearances similar to the glomerular filtration rate:**

    A   streptomycin
    B   penicillin
    C   chloramphenicol
    D   septrin
    E   gentamicin

    Your answers: A. . . . .B. . . . .C. . . . .D. . . . .E. . . . .

55. **Lignocaine**

    A   loses potency on repeat autoclaving
    B   causes methaemoglobinaemia
    C   causes convulsions
    D   must always be given with adrenaline in the treatment of dysrhythmias
    E   has a quinidide-like effect on A-V conduction

    Your answers: A. . . . .B. . . . .C. . . .D. . . . .E. . . . .

56. **Bronchodilation is brought about by**

    A   atropine
    B   methazolamide hydrochloride
    C   ephedrine
    D   tubocurarine
    E   oxprenolol

    Your answers: A. . . . .B. . . . .C. . . . .D. . . . .E. . . . .

57. Morphine

A causes spasm of the sphincter of Oddi
B raises arterial PCO_2
C increases ADH secretion
D decreases urinary sodium
E promotes histamine release

Your answers: A . . . . . B . . . . . C . . . . . D . . . . . E . . . . .

58. Involuntary movements occur with

A ketamine
B droperidol
C diazepam
D enflurane
E metoclopramide overdose

Your answers: A . . . . . B . . . . . C . . . . . D . . . . . E . . . . .

59. The effects of intravenous oxytocin given quickly include

A abdominal cramps
B hypertension
C arrhythmias
D nausea
E few side effects

Your answers: A . . . . . B . . . . . C . . . . . D . . . . . E . . . . .

60. Propranolol

A causes bronchodilation
B increases total peripheral resistance
C causes retention of urine
D is a negative inotrope
E blocks secretion of renin

Your answers: A . . . . . B . . . . . C . . . . . D . . . . . E . . . . .

61. Suxamethonium

A   is a quaternary amine
B   is similar in structure to acetylcholine
C   is metabolised by acetylcholinesterase
D   is potentiated by neostigmine
E   is stable in solution

Your answers: A.....B.....C.....D.....E.....

62. Isoflurane

A   causes greater respiratory depression than halothane
B   has a low blood gas solubility
C   causes cerebral vasodilation
D   is a halogenated methyl ethyl ether
E   sensitises the myocardium to catecholamines

Your answers: A.....B.....C.....D.....E.....

63. Drug metabolism in the liver

A   shortens the duration of action of highly ionised compounds
B   always reduces potency
C   is unaffected by hepatic blood flow
D   may involve combination with cytochrome P450
E   is influenced by polygenic inheritance

Your answers: A.....B.....C.....D.....E.....

64. The butyrophenones

A   inhibit the action of apomorphine at the chemoreceptor trigger zone
B   inhibit the action of atropine at vagal nerve endings
C   can produce hallucinations
D   give rise to marked respiratory depression
E   have a low incidence of extrapyramidal symptoms

Your answers: A.....B.....C.....D.....E.....

65. **Diazoxide**

    A   is related to the thiazides
    B   is an antihypertensive
    C   causes hypoglycaemia
    D   is an alpha blocker
    E   releases histamine

    Your answers: A.....B.....C.....D.....E.....

66. **The following are positive inotropes:**

    A   glucagon
    B   acetylcholine
    C   adrenaline
    D   isoprenaline
    E   ephedrine

    Your answers: A.....B.....C.....D.....E.....

67. **The following drugs are monoamine oxidase inhibitors:**

    A   phenylzine
    B   transcypramine
    C   amitriptyline
    D   imipramine
    E   flupenthixol

    Your answers: A.....B.....C.....D.....E.....

68. **Clonidine**

    A   is an α_2 agonist
    B   causes rebound hypertension on stopping treatment
    C   causes a tachycardia
    D   converts angiotensin 1
    E   is an α_1 antagonist

    Your answers: A.....B.....C.....D.....E.....

69. **The following drugs have been implicated in causing malignant hyperpyrexia:**

    A   suxamethonium
    B   β-blockers
    C   isoflurane
    D   nitrous oxide
    E   fentanyl

    Your answers: A. . . . .B. . . . .C. . . . .D. . . . .E. . . . .

70. **The following block neuronal monoamine uptake:**

    A   imipramine
    B   dopamine
    C   amitriptyline
    D   carbamizole
    E   isocarboxazid

    Your answers: A. . . . .B. . . . .C. . . . .D. . . . .E. . . . .

71. **The hypnotic effect of a given dose of a barbiturate is likely to be**

    A   prolonged if the drug is highly lipid soluble
    B   greater in epileptic subjects
    C   diminished by the simultaneous consumption of an alcoholic drink
    D   potentiated by hypoalbuminaemia
    E   reduced by alkalinisation of the urine

    Your answers: A. . . . .B. . . . .C. . . . .D. . . . .E. . . . .

72. **Plasma cholinesterase**

    A   is secreted by the reticuloendothelial system
    B   will hydrolyse benzoyl-choline
    C   is inhibited by sodium fluoride
    D   is found in erythrocytes
    E   can be congenitally absent

    Your answers: A. . . . .B. . . . .C. . . . .D. . . . .E. . . . .

73. **Salbutamol**

    A   is absorbed into the systemic circulation when administered by aerosol
    B   reduces pulmonary artery pressure
    C   is a bronchodilator
    D   causes tachycardia
    E   relaxes the pregnant uterus

    Your answers: A.....B.....C.....D.....E.....

74. **The following intravenous agents are dissolved in water for clinical use:**

    A   propanidid
    B   ketamine
    C   althesin
    D   etomidate
    E   suxamethonium

    Your answers: A.....B.....C.....D.....E.....

75. **Metoclopramide**

    A   increases prolactin secretion
    B   causes hypertension
    C   causes oculogyric crisis
    D   increases lower oesophageal tone
    E   causes nausea

    Your answers: A.....B.....C.....D.....E.....

76. **The following drugs may cause a tachycardia:**

    A   atropine
    B   fentanyl
    C   pancuronium
    D   gallamine
    E   vecuronium

    Your answers: A.....B.....C.....D.....E.....

77. Convulsions can be brought about by large doses of the following drugs/agents:

A   lignocaine
B   insulin
C   oxygen
D   nikethamide
E   amphetamine

Your answers: A.....B.....C.....D.....E.....

78. Naloxone

A   is a kappa agonist
B   is a mu agonist
C   reverses morphine induced vomiting
D   increases the blood pressure in hypovolaemic shock
E   reverses the action of pentazocine

Your answers: A.....B.....C.....D.....E.....

79. Isoflurane

A   does not sensitise the heart to catecholamines
B   has a minimum alveolar concentration (MAC) of 0.75
C   only 0.2% is metabolised in the liver
D   has little effect on overall systemic vascular resistance
E   preserves the liver blood flow

Your answers: A.....B.....C.....D.....E.....

80. Labetolol

A   is a β receptor agonist
B   is an α_2
C   antagonises angiotensin
D   its β effects are longer lasting than its α effects
E   it prevents release of noradrenaline from adrenergic nerve terminals

Your answers: A.....B.....C.....D.....E.....

PRACTICE EXAM 4

80 Questions: time allowed 2 ³/₄ hours. Indicate your answers by putting T (True) or F (False) in the spaces provided.

1. **Gastrin release is**

   A stimulated by partially digested meat in the stomach
   B stimulated by distension of the antrum of the stomach
   C followed by an increase in gastric blood flow
   D inhibited by vagal stimulation
   E inhibited by HCl in the stomach

   Your answers: A.....B.....C.....D.....E.....

2. **The bicarbonate buffer system is the most effective acid base buffer of**

   A interstitial fluid
   B erythrocytes
   C cerebrospinal fluid
   D cells of tissues
   E urine

   Your answers: A.....B.....C.....D.....E.....

3. **Factors increasing cardiac output are**

   A pyrexia
   B elevation of the legs
   C pressure within the abdomen
   D contraction of skeletal muscle
   E opening the chest as in thoracic surgery

   Your answers: A.....B.....C.....D.....E.....

4. **Oxygen therapy is of limited value in**

   A stagnant hypoxia
   B histotoxic hypoxia
   C anaemic hypoxia
   D in respiratory acidosis
   E hypoxic hypoxia due to shunting of unoxygenated venous blood past the lungs

   Your answers: A.....B.....C.....D.....E.....

63

5. Assuming that the condition is uncomplicated by any other disease, ankle oedema is seen in

A   renal failure
B   Kwashiorkor
C   heart failure
D   myxoedema
E   hypertension

Your answers: A. . . . .B. . . . .C. . . . .D. . . . .E. . . . .

6. Basal metabolic rate

A   is 170 kJ (40 kcal) per m^2 per hour
B   may be measured using an ergometer
C   is high in tropical climates
D   is low in children
E   is always elevated in patients with goitre

Your answers: A. . . . .B. . . . .C. . . . .D. . . . .E. . . . .

7. Measurement of airway resistance may entail the use of

A   an oesophageal balloon
B   body plethysmography
C   a pneumotachograph
D   a stethograph
E   a Haldane alveolar tube

Your answers: A. . . . .B. . . . .C. . . . .D. . . . .E. . . . .

8. Iron absorption

A   occurs most rapidly in the terminal ileum
B   is aided by HCl
C   depends on total body vitamin C
D   is active
E   is influenced by the total body iron

Your answers: A. . . . .B. . . . .C. . . . .D. . . . .E. . . . .

9. **The increase in myocardial wall thickness in left ventricular hypertrophy**

   A   is caused by an increase in the number of myocardial cells
   B   can occur in healthy subjects
   C   can occur as an adaptive response to systemic hypertension
   D   predisposes the subject to angina
   E   can be diagnosed by a large p wave in the ECG

   Your answers: A. . . . .B. . . . .C. . . . .D. . . . .E. . . .

10. **In a recumbent subject the greatest drop in blood pressure occurs between**

   A   the ascending aorta and brachial artery
   B   the saphenous vein and right atrium
   C   the femoral artery and femoral vein
   D   the arterial and venous ends of a capillary
   E   the pulmonary artery and left atrium

   Your answers: A. . . . .B. . . . .C. . . . .D. . . . .E. . . . .

11. **In the proximal convoluted tubule of the kidney**

   A   the fluid is hypotonic
   B   potassium ions are secreted
   C   PAH is actively secreted
   D HCO_3 is mainly absorbed in the form of CO_2
   E   chloride is actively reabsorbed

   Your answers: A. . . . .B. . . . .C. . . . .D. . . . .E. . . . .

12. **After surgical hypophysectomy for pituitary tumours the following may occur:**

   A   meningitis
   B   diabetes insipidus
   C   disturbances of reproductive function
   D   diabetes mellitus
   E   cerebrospinal fluid rhinorrhoea

   Your answers: A. . . . .B. . . . .C. . . . .D. . . . .E. . . . .

13. Photochemical dark adaptation

A occurs more rapidly in the cones than in the rods
B involves combination of opsin with 11-cis-retinal
C results when pigment cells lose their melanin
D does not occur in the fovea since inner retinal layers are absent
E occurs to a greater extent in rods than cones

Your answers: A.....B.....C.....D.....E.....

14. In the new born

A cardiac output is about 1 l/min at birth
B the glomerular filtration rate is about half that of the adult on a weight basis
C compared with the adult the kidney has a reduced osmolality and this is exacerbated in the premature newborn
D the alveolar ventilation is about twice that of the adult on a weight basis
E vasopressin is not secreted until about the 4th week and hence hypotonic urine is produced

Your answers: A.....B.....C.....D.....E.....

15. Coronary circulation

A shows vasoconstriction in hypotension
B flow is decreased in bradycardia
C shows vasodilatation on injection of adrenaline
D flow is increased in congestive heart failure
E flow in the left coronary artery is decreased during isometric relaxation of the ventricles

Your answers: A.....B.....C.....D.....E.....

16. Concerning oxygen consumption in the adult and its measurement

A using a spirometer entails measurement of the rate of emptying of the spirometer bell
B at rest the oxygen consumption is about 500 ml/min
C the consumption of one litre of oxygen is approximately equal to the production of 40 kJ (960 kcal)
D if the subject hyperventilates, the oxygen in the expired air will increase
E during moderate exercise ventilation increases linearly as oxygen consumption increases

Your answers: A.....B.....C.....D.....E.....

17. **Substances which become uniformly distributed through the body are**

    A   urea
    B   potassium
    C   Evans blue
    D   insulin
    E   deuterium oxide

    Your answers: A.....B.....C.....D.....E.....

18. **The term myogenic tone describes**

    A   the continuous activity in the sympathetic vasomotor system
    B   the continuous discharge of the annulo-spiral endings in muscle spindles
    C   the sustained contraction seen in smooth muscles
    D   the sustained contraction seen in postural skeletal muscles
    E   the sustained contraction seen in the absence of electrical activity in any muscle cell

    Your answers: A.....B.....C.....D.....E.....

19. **Erythropoietin**

    A   production is increased by a high $PaCO_2$
    B   is increased on hypoxia
    C   enhances proliferation of erythrocyte precursor cells
    D   is a polypeptide
    E   is produced in the bone marrow

    Your answers: A.....B.....C.....D.....E.....

20. **Oxygen availability to organs depends on**

    A   the tissue blood flow
    B   the haemoglobin concentration
    C   the PaO_2 of the blood
    D   the capillary blood flow
    E   mean arterial blood pressure

    Your answers: A.....B.....C.....D.....E.....

21. **When positive pressure respiration is used the patient is subjected to**

    A   increased cardiac output
    B   decreased venous return during the inspiratory positive pressure phase
    C   high blood pressure
    D   the same changes as encountered using hyperbaric oxygen
    E   aided expiration

    Your answers: A.....B.....C.....D.....E.....

22. **Following resection of the terminal ileum there is**

    A   megaloblastic anaemia due to vitamin B_{12} deficiency
    B   anaemia resulting from iron deficiency
    C   night blindness due to vitamin A deficiency
    D   steatorrhoea
    E   bleeding tendency due to vitamin K deficiency

    Your answers: A.....B.....C.....D.....E.....

23. **Parathyroid hormone secretion is increased**

    A   in vitamin D overdosage
    B   when the blood phosphate level falls
    C   in chronic renal failure
    D   on prolonged immobilisation in bed
    E   with acute decrease in plasma magnesium

    Your answers: A.....B.....C.....D.....E.....

24. **Retraction of the clot is most dependent on**

    A   the concentration of factor VIII
    B   leucocyte concentration
    C   the number of disintegrated platelets
    D   erythrocytes
    E   the number of intact platelets

    Your answers: A.....B.....C.....D.....E.....

25. The following are derived from the neural crest:

A   adrenal medulla
B   adrenal cortex
C   the pigment cells in the skin
D   Schwann cells along nerve axons
E   pigmented retina

Your answers: A.....B.....C.....D.....E.....

26. A unilateral pneumothorax results in

A   an increase in pulmonary residual volume
B   a collapse of the chest wall inward
C   a decrease in the intrapleural pressure (i.e. less negative)
D   a decrease in resting tidal volume
E   a shift in the mediastinum towards the normal side

Your answers: A.....B.....C.....D.....E.....

27. A low plasma potassium level

A   is caused by aldosterone deficiency
B   is an indication of depleted body potassium
C   is associated with prolonged vomiting of gastric contents
D   causes reduced intestinal peristalsis
E   can be associated with cardiac arrythmias

Your answers: A.....B.....C.....D.....E.....

28. A urinary output of 270 ml in the 24 h following an abdominal aortic aneurysm is suggestive of renal failure if

A   urine osmolality is 290 mOsm/kg
B   blood urea is 50 mmol/l
C   urinary urea is 350 mmol/l
D   serum bicarbonate is 30 mmol/l
E   plasma potassium is 7.5 mmol

Your answers: A.....B.....C.....D.....E.....

29. **As anaesthesia deepens**

    A   spontaneous ventilation ceases when the peripheral chemo-
        receptors cease responding
    B   a progressive fall in pH may occur
    C   the respiratory response to hypercapnia decreases
    D   the respiratory response to hypoxia is more affected than the
        response to hypercapnia
    E   carbon dioxide retention occurs

    Your answers: A.....B.....C.....D.....E.....

30. **Haemoglobin**

    A   in the fetus is produced primarily in the liver after the third
        month
    B   is only produced in bone marrow towards term
    C   is produced in the femur of a healthy adult man
    D   is produced in the vertebrae of a healthy adult
    E   is produced in the sternum of a healthy adult

    Your answers: A.....B.....C.....D.....E.....

31. **Secretion of androgens in the adult female**

    A   is not normally observed
    B   from an androgen secreting tumour does not affect the pitch of
        the voice
    C   from an androgen secreting tumour may result in amenorrhoea
    D   normally has no effect
    E   from an androgen secreting tumour may result in enlargement
        of the clitoris

    Your answers: A.....B.....C.....D.....E.....

32. **Section of the vagal nerves to the gastro-intestinal tract produces**

    A   decreased salivation
    B   decreased transit time
    C   decreased gastrin release
    D   increased gastric motility
    E   increased protein reabsorption

    Your answers: A.....B.....C.....D.....E.....

33. **Endocrine abnormalities associated with cirrhosis of the liver include**

   A   raised prolactin levels
   B   raised thyroxine levels due to diminished hormone conjugation
   C   raised plasma vasopressin
   D   abnormal thyroxine binding
   E   raised plasma aldosterone concentrations

   Your answers: A.....B.....C.....D.....E.....

34. **If the myelin surrounding a peripheral motor nerve is removed then**

   A   the potassium will seep away
   B   conduction will be slower than in a similar myelinated nerve
   C   nodes of Ranvier will be absent
   D   the axons will enlarge
   E   conduction may pass laterally from one demyelinated axon to another

   Your answers: A.....B.....C.....D.....E.....

35. **During pregnancy**

   A   upward displacement of the diaphragm reduces vital capacity
   B   the PCO_2 increases stimulating respiration
   C   the alveolar ventilation increases
   D   the increased progesterone concentrations influence the PCO_2
   E   the Bohr shift in the maternal blood aids in transfer of oxygen to the fetus

   Your answers: A.....B.....C.....D.....E.....

36. **Blood viscosity**

   A   increases exponentially with increasing packed cell volume
   B   decreases in tubes of very small diameter
   C   is increased in burns
   D   increases with higher velocities of blood flow
   E   is markedly affected even by small variations in plasma proteins

   Your answers: A.....B.....C.....D.....E.....

37. Concerning calcium in excitable tissues

A at rest it is present in higher concentrations in the cytoplasm of nerve and muscle cells than in the extracellular fluid

B a reduction in extracellular calcium concentrations decreases excitability

C an increase in extracellular calcium concentration results in enhanced neurotransmitter release

D provides a link between excitation and contraction in all muscle types

E an increase in extracellular calcium results in an increase in the strength of contraction of skeletal muscle fibres

Your answers: A.....B.....C.....D.....E.....

38. Complications of partial removal of the stomach include

A loss of weight

B malabsorption of fat

C constipation resulting from the loss of the gastro-colic reflex

D anaemia resulting from reduced vitamin B_6 absorption

E anaemia resulting from reduced reduction of the ferric to the ferrous form

Your answers: A.....B.....C.....D.....E.....

39. In the thyroid

A thyroid stimulating antibody resembles TRH in its actions

B thiocyanate competitively inhibits iodide uptake

C thiouracil inhibits oxidation of iodide to iodine and the synthesis of thyroxine

D the output of T3 is greater than T4

E iodide enters against an electric gradient

Your answers: A.....B.....C.....D.....E.....

40. Respiratory minute work is increased by

A airway constriction

B disappearance of turbulence

C increased density of the inspired gas

D increased compliance of the lungs

E increased tidal volume

Your answers: A.....B.....C.....D.....E.....

41. **Vasopressin**

    A decreases the permeability of the collecting ducts of the kidney
    B acts by increasing intracellular cyclic AMP
    C is released in response to neural impulses originating in the hypothalamus
    D is secreted in response to hypovolaemia
    E secretion is enhanced in response to pain

    Your answers: A.....B.....C.....D.....E.....

42. **Activation of parasympathetic nerve fibres results in**

    A defaecation
    B micturition
    C sweating
    D ejaculation of semen
    E dilation of the pupil

    Your answers: A.....B.....C.....D.....E.....

43. **Treatment with an aldosterone antagonist may result in a fall in**

    A urine volume
    B blood volume
    C packed cell volume
    D plasma potassium concentrations
    E plasma osmolality

    Your answers: A.....B.....C.....D.....E.....

44. **Oversecretion from the adrenal cortex (Cushing's syndrome) is likely to result in**

    A puffiness of the face and abdomen
    B redistribution of body mass from limbs to trunk
    C raised blood sugar
    D hypertrophy of skeletal muscles
    E reduction of plasma K^+ concentration

    Your answers: A.....B.....C.....D.....E.....

45. **The standard deviation (SD) of a series of observations**

A gives an indication of the scatter of the observations
B should only be calculated if the observations have a normal distribution
C indicates the significance of the observations
D may be given by the formula $\dfrac{\sqrt{\varepsilon(x-\bar{x})^2}}{n}$ where x is the mean of n observations
E may be calculated with a variation of the formula given in D

Your answers: A.....B.....C.....D.....E.....

46. **Isoprenaline**

A can be given sublingually
B is absorbed from the stomach
C is blocked by phenothiazines
D is worse than adrenaline in producing cardiac dysrhythmias
E is absorbed if administered via an aerosol

Your answers: A.....B.....C.....D.....E.....

47. **The following drugs pass readily through the blood brain barrier:**

A levodopa
B hyoscine
C hyoscine-N-butyl bromide
D paracetamol
C 5-hydroxytryptamine

Your answers: A.....B.....C.....D.....E.....

48. **Propofol**

A is dissolved in 10% soya bean oil fat emulsion
B decreases blood pressure as a result of vasodilatation
C is broken down by plasma cholinesterase
D a sleep dose is 4–5 mg/kg in a healthy unpremedicated adult
E is more respiratory depressant than thiopentone

Your answers: A.....B.....C.....D.....E.....

49. **The following are potassium sparing diuretics:**

A chlorthiazide
B spironolactone
C frusemide
D mannitol
E acetazolamide

Your answers: A.....B.....C.....D.....E.....

50. **The hypoglycaemic effects of chlorpropamide may**

A occur more than 24 hours after the last dose
B be exaggerated by sulphonamides
C be inhibited by phenylbutazone
D be undetected if the patient is taking propranolol
E be increased by thiazide diuretics

Your answers: A.....B.....C.....D.....E.....

51. **The following drugs are made more active by metabolism:**

A dichloralphenazone
B paracetamol
C caffeine
D prednisone
E phenytoin

Your answers: A.....B.....C.....D.....E.....

52. **Which of the following antagonises insulin:**

A diazoxide
B glucagon
C adrenaline
D propranolol
E tolbutamide

Your answers: A.....B.....C.....D.....E.....

53. **Methohexitone differs from thiopentone in that methohexitone**

A   is metabolised more rapidly
B   is comprised of two isomers
C   can be used in porphyria
D   causes less excitation phenomena
E   is a thiobarbiturate

Your answers: A. . . . .B. . . . .C. . . .D. . . .E. . . . .

54. **Neostigmine**

A   is a competitive inhibitor of acetylcholinesterase
B   has a direct effect on the binding of the nondepolarising muscle
     relaxant with the receptor site
C   causes bronchodilation
D   increases intestinal peristalsis
E   will always reverse prolonged suxamethonium block

Your answers: A. . . . .B. . . . .C. . . .D. . . .E. . . . .

55. **Jaundice has been associated with the following agents:**

A   diethyl ether
B   trichloroethylene
C   halothane
D   chloroform
E   methoxyflurane

Your answers: A. . . . .B. . . . .C. . . .D. . . .E. . . . .

56. **Alveolar concentration of a volatile agent approaches the inspired concentration faster if**

A   inspired concentration is increased
B   ventilation is increased
C   the agent is more potent
D   the mixed venous tension is increased
E   nitrous oxide is added

Your answers: A. . . . .B. . . . .C. . . .D. . . .E. . . . .

57. **In non-depolarising neuromuscular block**

    A fasciculation occurs prior to blockade
    B neostigmine acts by inhibiting the breakdown of acetylcholine
    C partial block is indicated by post tetanic facilitation
    D is always prolonged by metabolic acidosis
    E is prolonged by concurrent administration of aminoglycoside antibiotics

    Your answers: A.....B.....C.....D.....E.....

58. **The following affect the placental transfer of lignocaine:**

    A the placental blood flow
    B pH
    C plasma protein binding
    D extent of foetal liver metabolism of lignocaine
    E lipid solubility

    Your answers: A.....B.....C.....D.....E.....

59. **Aminoglycosides in overdosage can cause**

    A bone marrow suppression
    B tinnitus
    C neuromuscular block
    D polyuric renal failure
    E ataxia

    Your answers: A.....B.....C.....D.....E.....

60. **Pentazocine**

    A is more potent than morphine
    B is a respiratory depressant
    C can be reversed by naloxone
    D can cause hallucinations
    E is a partial agonist

    Your answers: A.....B.....C.....D.....E.....

61. Atropine

A causes more sedation than hyoscine
B has a greater cardiac effect than hyoscine
C has a greater antisialogogue effect than glycopyrrolate
D in overdosage can cause hyperpyrexia
E completely blocks all the actions of acetylcholine

Your answers: A.....B.....C.....D.....E.....

62. Acetylcholine receptors are blocked by

A trimetaphan
B hexamethonium
C ouabain
D diphenylhydramine
E benzhexol

Your answers: A.....B.....C.....D.....E.....

63. Dopamine

A is an antagonist
B increases mesenteric blood flow
C increases renal blood flow
D is a positive inotrope
E decreases the peripheral to central temperature gradient

Your answers: A.....B.....C.....D.....E.....

64. Cimetidine

A is an H_1 antagonist
B crosses the placenta
C reduces gastric acidity
D inhibits cytochrome P450
E relaxes the uterus

Your answers: A.....B.....C.....D.....E.....

65. **Digoxin can be used in**

A atrial flutter
B idioventricular rhythms
C ventricular tachycardia
D cardiac tamponade
E 2:1 block

Your answers: A.....B.....C.....D.....E.....

66. **The following are anti-emetics:**

A hyoscine
B carbimazole
C perphenazine
D apomorphine
C cyclizine

Your answers: A.....B.....C.....D.....E.....

67. **Excretion of the following drugs is increased with an alkaline diuresis:**

A salicylates
B barbiturates
C pethidine
D tricyclics
E theophylline

Your answers: A.....B.....C.....D.....E.....

68. **The following drugs may accelerate labour:**

A salbutamol
B prostaglandin $F_2\alpha$
C acetyl salicylic acid
D oxytocin
E alcohol

Your answers: A.....B.....C.....D.....E.....

69. **Methohexitone**

   A is a thiobarbiturate
   B is contraindicated in acute intermittent porphyria
   C is less potent than thiopentone
   D is protein bound
   E is excreted unchanged in the urine

   Your answers: A.....B.....C.....D.....E.....

70. **The following statements are true:**

   A enflurane is an alkane
   B methoxyflurane is a substituted methyl ethyl ether
   C isoflurane has a higher blood gas coefficient than halothane
   D isoflurane decreases systemic vascular resistance whereas halothane does not
   E isoflurane is an isomer of enflurane

   Your answers: A.....B.....C.....D.....E.....

71. **Enzyme induction can be produced by**

   A chlorpromazine
   B DDT
   C phenobarbitone
   D diazepam
   E nitrazepam

   Your answers: A.....B.....C.....D.....E.....

72. **The following antibiotics give rise to satisfactory blood levels when taken by mouth:**

   A cephalothin
   B kanamycin
   C vancomycin
   D carbenicillin
   E flucloxacillin

   Your answers: A.....B.....C.....D.....E.....

73. **Placental transfer of a drug is less likely if**

    A   it is lipid soluble
    B   it has a molecular weight greater than 600
    C   it is metabolised slowly
    D   it is highly ionised
    E   it is administered in small doses

    Your answers: A.....B.....C.....D.....E.....

74. **Enflurane**

    A   is non explosive in air but explosive in oxygen
    B   has a low blood/gas coefficient
    C   has stimulant effects on the CNS and can cause convulsions
    D   is an isomer of isoflurane
    E   produces marked respiratory depression

    Your answers: A.....B.....C.....D.....E.....

75. **Nitrous oxide**

    A   is so rapidly taken up that Stage 111 anaesthesia is readily attained
    B   cylinders also contain small amounts of nitric oxide and nitrogen dioxide
    C   can give rise to bone marrow depression after prolonged exposure
    D   can give rise to methaemoglobinaemina after prolonged exposure
    E   lowers the MAC of concurrently administered inhalational agents

    Your answers: A.....B.....C.....D.....E.....

76. **Propofol**

    A   has a steroid structure
    B   has a pH greater than 10
    C   is prepared in aqueous emulsion
    D   is excreted unchanged in the urine
    E   may cause pain on injection

    Your answers: A.....B.....C.....D.....E.....

77. **Morphine**

    A releases histamine
    B increases gut motility
    C causes bronchoconstriction
    D raises the blood sugar
    E may be antagonised by pentazocine

    Your answers: A.....B.....C.....D.....E.....

78. **Propranolol**

    A is prepared as a racaemic mixture
    B slows A-V conduction
    C has local anaesthetic action
    D slows the upstroke of the action potential
    E causes bronchoconstriction

    Your answers: A.....B.....C.....D.....E.....

79. **The following drugs cross the placenta:**

    A neostigmine
    B curare
    C suxamethonium
    D hyoscine
    E thiopentone

    Your answers: A.....B.....C.....D.....E.....

80. **Muscle pains associated with the use of suxamethonium**

    A can be reduced by priming with a small dose of gallamine
    B can be abolished by using suxamethonium bromide
    C are more common in children and the elderly
    D are reduced by early post operative mobilisation
    E are related to the extent of muscle fasciculation

    Your answers: A.....B.....C.....D.....E.....

ANSWERS AND EXPLANATIONS

The correct answer options are given against each question.

1. **AC**
   Active transport involves the movement of a substance from a region of low concentration to one of higher concentration and necessitates the expenditure of energy. Two means of linking energy to the transport are known. Primary active transport involves the direct use of ATP, while secondary active transport employs a sodium concentration gradient to supply energy. Three primary active transport carriers have been identified, one pumping sodium and potassium, one calcium and one hydrogen. A hydrogen pump is involved in the production of HCl in the stomach. The sodium potassium pump contributes to the characteristic distribution of ions across cell membranes. Magnesium exists in higher concentrations in the cells than in the extracellular fluid and exits down the concentration gradient. Hormone secretion involves exocytosis for peptide hormones and tyrosine derivatives and diffusion for steroid hormones.

2. **ABE**
   Inherited defects of haemoglobin production fall into two groups. In the first group there is a qualitative change, usually resulting from a single amino acid substitution in one of the globin chains, as for sickle cell disease in which a valine is substituted for glutamic acid. The resulting haemoglobin, HbS, forms polymers when oxygen tension is reduced, which produces alteration in the shape of the red cell and an increase in the viscosity of the blood. The second type of disorder, the thalassaemias, is caused by quantitative changes in the amount of α or β haemoglobin production. In β-thalassaemia the normal haemoglobin, HbA, (α_2, β_2) is reduced and fetal haemoglobin, HbF, $(\alpha_2 \gamma_2)$ persists into adult life. If all the chains are deleted HbH is produced (β_4).

3. **D**
   The output of the heart per unit time is the cardiac output and in the resting male is about 5.5 l/min. The resting cardiac output is related to the surface area. The cardiac output per min per square metre of body surface is the cardiac index; it averages 3.2 l/min/m^2.

83

4. B

At altitude the barometric pressure falls, although the composition of the inspired air is essentially unaltered. The partial pressure of the inspired oxygen falls and therefore the alveolar PO_2 does also and the percent saturation of arterial blood with oxygen. The amount of water carried in the air depends on its temperature and since the temperature of the inspired air is constant at around 37°C, the saturated water vapour pressure remains constant at 47 mm Hg. The partial pressure of CO_2 also remains constant at around 40 mm Hg.

5. ACD

In renal disease the breakdown products of protein metabolism accumulate in the blood and uraemia develops. There is also a failure to excrete the acid products of digestion and metabolism such as the hydrogen and sulphate ions derived from sulphur containing amino acids and hydrogen and phosphate containing substances such as nucleoproteins. This results from metabolic failure, so hydrogen ions are not transported against the concentration gradient and there is an inadequate supply of ammonia. The fall in glomerular filtration rate results in a shortage of filtered buffer to make titrable acid.

6. BDE

Calcium is absorbed mainly in the duodenum and to some extent in the upper jejunum. Some passive diffusion occurs but absorption is largely an active process. The absorption may involve a calcium binding protein and it has also been suggested that a Ca-ATPase is involved. The synthesis of the calcium binding protein is induced by a metabolite of vitamin D. 1,25 dihydroxycholecalciferol under the influence of circulating parathyroid hormone. Calcium absorption is facilitated by lactose and protein and is inhibited by phosphate and oxalate because these form insoluble salts with calcium in the intestine.

7. CD

Upward displacement of the diaphragm might be expected to reduce vital capacity, but the diminished height of the pleural cavity is compensated by an increase in width. Thus vital capacity is unchanged. The increased ventilation is due to a greater sensitivity of the respiratory centre to CO_2 which results in a reduced $PaCO_2$. This may be an effect of the increased progesterone concentrations. Oxygen consumption is increased by about 18% during pregnancy mainly to satisfy the needs of the fetus.

8. E

When the motor nerve to a skeletal muscle is stimulated acetylcholine is released at the motor end plate. This leads to a surface membrane and then to a t-tubule action potential. The sarcoplasmic reticulum releases calcium which binds to troponin and via tropomyosin allows the actin and myosin to interact. The myosin 'heads' move along the actin. The speed of shortening is not proportional to the load opposing shortening. Heat as well as shortening is produced during muscle activity.

9. BE

Tendon reflexes are phasic reflexes and thus depend on the monosynaptic reflex arc. The reflex depends on the primary endings in the muscle spindle served by the fast conducting 1a afferent fibres which make monosynaptic connections with their own and with synergistic motor neurones and inhibitory connections with antagonistic motor neurones. The reflex is initiated by stretch of the muscle so that the term tendon reflex is misleading. The tendon organs are found in the junction of the tendon with the muscles and are supplied by 1b fibres. The muscle spindle mainly detects the length of the muscle, whereas tendon organs mainly measure tension. The knee jerk is effectively a spinal reflex, but both it and the ankle jerk are exaggerated in tetraplegics.

10. CE

Magnetic resonance imaging employs non-ionising radiofrequency radiation in the presence of a structured magnetic field. This is not a real time technique and therefore respiratory motion will lead to degradation of image quality. It can distinguish between different tissue types which is important, for example in endometrial cancer and in the differentiation of benign and malignant ovarian masses. It is not known to have adverse side effects. However imaging is not advised in the first three months of pregnancy.

11. CD

Determination of plasma volume depends on the dilution technique. A known amount of a harmless substance is injected and its concentration in the plasma determined after thorough mixing. Volume may then be determined:

Volume = Amount injected/Plasma concentration

This technique may be used to determine the volume of any body compartment. In order to be employed in the determination of

plasma volume the substance has to remain within the cardiovascular space and not penetrate the red cells. Such substances
include Evan's blue dye (T-1824) and radio-iodinated albumin.
Inulin and creatinine are employed to determine glomerular
filtration rate and para-amino hippuric acid to determine renal
plasma flow.

12. **AE**
The arterial pressure response to the Valsalva manoeuvre is used as
a test of ventricular function. The patient blows up a column of
mercury to 40 mm Hg and maintains the pressure for 10 sec. Initially
there is an increase in the intrathoracic pressure resulting in an
increase in blood pressure. The rise in intrathoracic pressure cuts
off the venous return to the right atrium so that the arterial pressure
falls as the central reservoir of blood in the heart and lung is
gradually emptied. The fall in arterial pressure initiates baroreceptor reflexes resulting in an increase in the peripheral resistance
and after a slight tachycardia a rise in the mean arterial pressure. On
releasing the pressure the cardiac output increases and given the
peripheral vasoconstriction there is an increase in blood pressure
which stimulates the baroreceptors and produces cardiac slowing,
the latter being the best sign of a normal clinical response.

13. **ABDE**
The carotid bodies contain clusters of two types of cells - type I cells
which are glomus cells surrounded by the type II cells. At intervals
between these cells are unmyelinated endings of the glossopharyngeal nerve fibres and it has been suggested that these are the
chemoreceptors which monitor oxygen tension. They are also
stimulated by hypercapnia and acidity. The blood flow is about 20
ml/g/min as compared to 0.54 ml/g/min in the brain. The flow is thus
so large so that there is little A-V difference and the capillary
oxygen tension is similar to the arterial. It also means that the
requirements of the tissue are met by dissolved oxygen so that
sensitivity is to the arterial PO_2 rather than the oxygen content.
Hence the receptors are not stimulated by conditions such as
anaemia and carbon monoxide poisoning. Changes in blood flow
alter the apparent sensitivity to arterial gases. For example a fall in
blood flow resulting from a fall in blood pressure stimulates the
carotid body with no changes in gas tensions.

14. **ABDE**
Absorption of the majority of filtered water and solutes takes place
in the proximal convoluted tubule. The tubular epithelium in this

region is quite permeable and the transtubular potential is only 3 mV. In contrast the distal tubule, where regulation of fluid balance occurs, is relatively impermeable. The loop of Henle is the region of the nephron where the concentration gradient is produced in the kidney. Production of the gradient depends on active pumping of sodium chloride in the thick ascending loop of Henle and the impermeability of the ascending limb of the loop of Henle to water. The vasa recta is permeable to water, the plasma becoming more concentrated as it approaches the tip of the loop of Henle.

15. BCD *1? Question mentions Percutereal Vit.k!*
In obstructive jaundice bile is excluded from the intestine. The absence of bile salts prevents vitamin K absorption as it is a fat soluble vitamin. The result is that prothrombin and factor VII are decreased and prothrombin time is prolonged. In severe cases clotting time may also be prolonged and haemorrhage may occur. The condition may be treated by giving bile salts alone, bile salts and vitamin K by mouth or more rapidly by injection of vitamin K given intramuscularly.

16. AB
The anterior pituitary hormone secretes the trophic hormones luteinising hormone (LH), follicular stimulating hormone (FSH), adrenocorticotrophic hormone (ACTH) and thyroid stimulating hormone (TSH), as well as growth hormone and prolactin. Oxytocin and vassopressin are released from the posterior pituitary. Release of trophic hormones is controlled by releasing and inhibiting hormones in the hypothalamus. Thyrotrophin releasing hormone is one such hormone.

17. ADE
Spermatozoa, being produced in the testes which lie outside the abdomen are below 37°C and spermatogenesis depends on a temperature about 4°C below body temperature. Both testosterone and FSH are necessary for normal spermatogenesis. Normal sperm are motile and can move at the rate of 1.0 mm/min which allows them to reach the oviduct within about 30 min. It is here that fertilisation takes place. Penetration of the zona pellucida that surrounds the ovum is facilitated by the release of acrosin a trypsin-like proteolytic enzyme.

18. ABC
Anaesthetic fluid injected around the stellate (cervico-thoracic) ganglion blocks transmission of stimuli through the cervical and

superior thoracic ganglia. This step is taken to relieve vascular spasms involving the brain and upper limbs. Stellate ganglion blockade removes the sympathetic supply to the head and neck on that side leading to vasodilatation of skin vessels and absence of sweating, constriction of the pupils, drooping of the upper lid (ptosis) and endophthalmos.

19. ABCDE

Triglycerides comprise more than 90% of dietary fat. Bile acids are necessary for absorption of fats. They act as detergents promoting emulsification of the fats, providing a greater surface area for the lipase to act. They also contribute to polymolecular aggregates, micelles, which serve to render substances, such as cholesterol, water soluble. The monoglycerides and fatty acids from the micelles are taken up into interstitial cells. Monoglycerides and fatty acids containing more than 14 carbon atoms are re-esterified to tri-glycerides which are then coated with lipoprotein to form chylo-microns. These enter the lymphatics which transport them to the thoracic duct and thence to the blood stream. When bile is excluded from the intestine as much as 25% of the dietary fat appears in the faeces.

20. D

At 20 kg a child may be anaesthetised with an anaesthetic machine used for adults. Lung compliance follows the size of the lungs. Thus compliance is high in the child and there is a fall in resistance as the child grows. The blood volume of a child this size is about 1.6l. The cardiac output is greater on a weight basis than in the adult and the blood pressure is 100/86. The GFR in the infant is less on a weight basis than that of the adult and progressively increases.

21. AD

The alveolar arterial gradient is the best single indicator of the exchange properties of the respiratory system. It depends largely on two factors. The first is the character of the membrane across which diffusion occurs and the second the physiological shunt. Breathing low oxygen has two effects; it increases the membrane component so that the alveolar mean capillary oxygen gradient becomes measurable, but greatly reduces the effect of the shunt component. The gradient is also affected by the cardiac output, which alters the transit time. The PaO_2 is not influenced by the haemoglobin carrying capacity.

22. **ADE**

Surface tension at an air liquid interface arises because the molecules of the liquid are drawn more into the liquid than the gas phase. The result is equivalent to a tension at the surface which leads to a decreased surface area. For pure liquids and true solutions the magnitude of this tension is a constant dependent upon the chemical nature of the gas and liquid involved and the temperature. As the temperature rises the surface tension falls. The surface tension of any liquid in contact with air is proportional to the fourth power of the density. If the surface is spherical then $T = P \times r/2$. Thus pressures are greater inside smaller bubbles than larger and so smaller alveoli would empty into larger were it not for the surfactant.

23. **ABD**

Inulin is used as a measure of glomerular filtration rate as the volume of plasma completely cleared of inulin per unit time equals the volume of plasma filtered per unit time. It is not bound to plasma protein and is freely filtered, but not reabsorbed or secreted. Furthermore it is not metabolised in the kidney and is biologically inert and non-toxic. Other substances such as mannitol, sorbitol and radio-labelled thyropaque may be used. Endogenous creatinine is used clinically to estimate glomerular filtration rate, but a small amount is secreted. Urea was at one time used, but urea clearance is only constant at flow rates above 2 ml/min. At normal urine flows urine excretion and hence clearance depends on the square root of urine flow.

24. **AE**

During starvation the individual must live on component tissues of the body, but although it may drop a little, blood glucose concentrations are maintained. The glycogen stores are called on, but are only several hundred grams. The main source of energy must be the fat reserves and tissue protein, but so long as fat is available, tissue is used sparingly. The fat is metabolised (lipolysis) and taken to the liver where it is completely dissimilated or transformed into ketone bodies which are sent to other tissues for oxidation. The ketones pass into the blood from the liver at a rate faster than they are disposed of by the tissue, so that ketosis results with acid urine containing ketone bodies. Plasma tri-iodothyronine is reduced so that there is a fall in basal metabolic rate and conservation of calories and protein.

25. BDE

Vasopressin, the antidiuretic hormone is synthesised in the magno-cellular neurones of the hypothalamus and released from the nerve terminals in the posterior pituitary. It appears that this final common pathway is stimulated by acetyl choline, nicotinic receptors being involved. The physiological stimuli for the release of the hormone are an increase in plasma osmolality and a fall in plasma volume. These two stimuli interact so that hypertonicity is a more effective stimulus in the presence of hypovolaemia and hypotension. Vasopressin acts on the collecting ducts to increase water permeability so that there is increased water retention and an antidiuresis.

26. ACDE

The muscle spindle, the sense organ of the muscle comprises 2–10 muscle fibres, which have a motor supply of their own. Thus if, for example, spindle muscle fibres contract during shortening of the skeletal muscle, the tension in the central region where the stretch receptors are located is maintained. The afferents are co-activated with motor neurones. It appears that motor neurones are activated according to the strength of the intended contraction and the afferents according to the distance of the intended movement. It seems that in most voluntary actions the efferents are of limited importance; they are probably of most importance when an action is learned. The efferent activity is believed to be important in the control of respiratory muscles. This is consistent with the observation that in most patients, in whom the cervical and thoracic dorsal roots were severed to alleviate pain caused by impenetrable tumours, less intercostal and/or diaphragmatic activity occurred.

27. AE

Provided the same stimulus strength is being used, the same number of fibres are activated as in a single twitch. In a fused tetanus the duration of the action potential of the muscle is less than the stimulus interval. A pulse of calcium is released from the sarco-plasmic reticulum following each action potential and if this is not fully absorbed by the time of the next action potential, the calcium concentration will sum. The tension developed depends on the level of the cytoplasmic calcium.

28. ABC

Cerebral blood flow may be estimated using the Fick principle. An agent employed is 15% nitrous oxide in an oxygen/nitrogen mixture, which the subject breathes for 15 min. Blood samples are removed from the internal jugular bulb and a peripheral artery. The cerebral blood flow in ml/100g/minute is then given by

$$\text{Flow} = \frac{\text{Amount of } N_2O \text{ taken up by the brain}}{(A\text{-}V) \ N_2O \text{ concentration}}$$

The cerebral blood flow is approximately 50 ml/100g/min. Cerebral autoregulation occurs, but the mechanism is believed to be chiefly metabolic; as the perfusing pressure decreases CO_2 accumulation produces vasodilatation through its conversion to hydrogen ions. Cerebral hypoxia will also cause release of pyruvic and lactic acids. Cerebral blood flow is greater through the region of the cells (grey matter) than around the axons (white matter).

29. CD
Amongst its various functions, the cerebrospinal fluid (c.s.f.) maintains a constant ionic environment in the brain and contributes to the control of respiration and pH. Approximately 70% of the c.s.f. is derived from the choroid plexus in networks of blood vessels covered with ependyma projecting into the ventricles. The remaining 30% comes from endothelial cells lining brain capillaries. The composition of the c.s.f. reveals that it is not merely an ultrafiltrate of plasma; there is active transport of sodium ions via $Na^+ K^+$ ATPase and chloride via the carbonic anhydrase system. The PCO_2 in the c.s.f. of about 50 mm Hg is higher than in arterial blood and the pH is about 7.33. The sodium concentration is approximately the same in plasma and c.s.f., but the chloride is present in slightly greater concentrations and the glucose in considerably lower.

30. ABDE
Cell membranes comprise a bilayer of lipids largely composed of cholesterol and phospholipids with proteins spanning the bilayer. Water is transported across this membrane, the driving force being osmotic pressure. Water, like urea and ions, penetrates the cells via water filled pores. Water crosses membranes relatively rapidly, some 10–100 times faster than urea and faster than methanol which has higher lipid solubility and would be expected to cross more rapidly. Membranes also show ion selectivity, so that the human erythrocyte membrane is far more permeable to chloride ions than potassium, whereas potassium and chloride permeate equally well in the resting muscle. Sodium is always pumped across a gradient. Glucose crosses the membrane via a carrier mediated process.

31. C

The total dead space represents the volume of the conducting system of airways, namely the anatomical dead space together with the alveoli which are ventilated but not perfused. In measuring the dead space with Fowler's method 100% oxygen is inspired at the end of a normal inspiration so that the dead space is filled with oxygen. The partial pressure of nitrogen is measured on expiration. It is initially zero, rising to plateau as the supplemental oxygen is washed out. The volume of air expired at the mid point of the initial rising phase of nitrogen tension represents the volume of the dead space.

32. ABC

The effect of gravity means that lung ventilation and perfusion are posture dependent. The arterial pressure and hence perfusion increases in the lower parts of the lung due to the hydrostatic effect. Ventilation also increases in the lower parts of the lung. Because of the weight of the lung the intrapleural pressure is greater at the bottom than at the top. The regional differences in intrapleural pressure gives rise to regional differences in ventilation because the relation between the increase in volume and pressure is not linear. Thus for a given expanding force the lower part of the lung fills more easily. There is a greater change in the perfusion rate than ventilation so that the ventilation perfusion ratio is higher on the dependent side. When the Va/Q increases the alveolar partial pressure of oxygen rises and the partial pressure of carbon dioxide falls. *Acc. to WEST D are are correct as well*

33. ADE

Normally when a limb is moved to stretch the muscle, there is mild resistance to the passive movement referred to as muscle tone. Tone is in part due to the intrinsic elasticity of the tissue, but is also the result of the activation of motor units with stretch of the muscle spindles. An increase in the input of the alpha and gamma motor neurones results in an increase in muscle tone (hypertonia). A reduction in either the afferent input from the muscle spindles or the efferent activity of the lower motor neurone results in a decrease of muscle tone (hypotonia).

34. BE

The blood flow varies in different parts of the lung because of the low pressure head, the distensibility of the vessels and the hydrostatic effects of gravity. Pulmonary vessels are plentifully supplied with sympathetic vasoconstrictor nerves and it has been demonstrated that, for example, chemoreceptor stimulation produces reflex pulmonary vasoconstriction. Despite this fact, it appears that regulation of overall pulmonary blood flow is largely passive and local adjustments of perfusion to ventilation are determined by the local PO_2. The pulmonary vessels are very distensible so that in exercise increases in transmural pressure produce dilatation which reduces resistance to flow. Exercise is also associated with opening of previously closed portions of the vascular bed. A survey of the blood flow can be performed by giving 133Xe intravenously while monitoring the chest. The gas rapidly enters the alveoli that are perfused normally, but fails to enter those that are not perfused.

35. AE

On submersion in water for every 10 m ($=$ 33 ft) the pressure increases by one atmosphere. Therefore at 30 m the pressure is 3 atmospheres above normal giving a total pressure of 4 atmospheres. The ambient pressure increase results in an elevated PO_2 to 56 kPa (400 mm Hg). Since Boyle's law ($PV=K$) holds for all air filled cavities the lung volume decreases approaching that near maximal expiration, the minimum volume being reached between 30 and 40 m. Because the lung volume cannot be further compressed at greater depths the intrathoracic pressure remains constant. The resulting pressure difference causes a considerable inflow of blood into the thoracic organs. Nitrogen at a pressure of greater than 4 atmospheres produces narcosis. Pressures less than this present no problems at depth, but as the diver ascends, nitrogen which tends to dissolve in the body, especially fat, comes out of solution and if the ascent is rapid will form tiny bubbles causing decompression sickness.

36. ABC

The CO_2 response curve is a plot of ventilation (in litres) against alveolar PCO_2 in the presence of a constant alveolar PO_2. The slope of the CO_2 response curve increases when the alveolar PO_2 is decreased. Thus when an individual is hypoxic they are more sensitive to increased arterial PCO_2. Even though the slope may change the intercept stays constant just below the normal alveolar PCO_2. There is a slight CO_2 drive of the respiratory centre. In contrast to the effect of oxygen, the hydrogen ion effects are additive with those of carbon dioxide so that during acidosis the CO_2 response curves are shifted to the left.

37. ADE

The Frank-Starling law states that the energy of contractility is proportional to the initial length of the cardiac muscle fibre. This effect is important in balancing the output of the two sides of the heart over an extended period. The relationship may be demonstrated in an innervated heart and stimulation of sympathetic or parasympathetic nerves shifts the curve of the relationship between the end diastolic volume and stroke volume. Starling's law predicts that a fully functional heart is small at rest and when a load is imposed enlarges in response to increased venous return. However on exercise the reverse occurs. This results from the increased contractility resulting from sympathetic stimulation. Thus Starling's mechanism does operate in man, but may be masked.

38. ABDE

Because of the effect of gravity, the mean arterial blood pressure in the feet of a normal adult is 180–200 mm Hg and the venous pressure is 85–90 mm Hg. The result is that blood tends to pool in the capacitance vessels of the lower extremities. However compensatory mechanisms are triggered by the fall in blood pressure in the carotid sinus and aortic arch resulting in a fall in baroreceptor activity. This reflexly leads to an increase in heart rate which helps to maintain the cardiac output despite the fall in stroke volume. Maintenance of blood volume is aided by arteriolar constriction. Thus there is a fall in abdominal and limb flows.

39. BDE

Three hormones can influence plasma calcium concentrations, namely parathyroid hormone, calcitonin and vitamin D. Vitamin D is essential for bone calcification. Failure to calcify bone results in an excess of osteoid tissue in uncalcified bone matrix. In very high doses, vitamin D can elevate plasma calcium independently of parathyroid hormone. Alkaline phosphatase is elevated in cholestatic jaundice and sometimes in liver disease, but does not reflect osteoclastic activity. Calcitonin lowers plasma calcium, but has little effect in man.

40. BCD

Blood sugar is elevated with insufficient endocrine secretion from the pancreas. The exocrine secretion contains bicarbonate which neutralises gastric acid and regulates the pH of the upper intestine. It also contains enzymes which digest the three major types of food, protein, carbohydrate and fat. Pancreatic enzymes are especially important in the digestion of protein and fats and if inadequate, protein digestion would be impaired. Fat digestion would be similarly impaired and, as a result, also the absorption of the fat soluble vitamins K and D. Vitamin K is important for normal production of prothrombin and factors VII, IX and X.

41. **ABCD**
Insulin acts to reduce blood glucose concentrations. Insulin action is antagonised by a number of factors including the hormones adrenaline, glucagon, cortisol, growth hormone, oestrogens, thyroid hormones and prolactin (in pregnancy); also insulin antibodies, plasma protein antagonists and an increase in free fatty acids. The autonomic nervous system is involved in insulin secretion and the β-adrenergic blocking agent propranolol inhibits insulin release. Biguanides lower blood glucose in diabetics. They do not cause hypoglycaemia in normal adults and are inactive in the absence of insulin.

42. **ABD**
The autonomic nervous system comprises sympathetic and parasympathetic systems. Preganglionic fibres of the sympathetic system have cell bodies in the thoracic and upper lumbar segments. The axons pass out of the spinal cord in the ventral roots. On leaving the spinal column preganglionic fibres form the white rami communicantes and join a distinct group of sympathetic ganglia, the vertebral (paravertebral or chain) ganglia. The postganglionic sympathetic nerves to the head originate in the superior and middle cervical stellate ganglia in the cranial extension of the sympathetic ganglion chain. The preganglionic nerves of the parasympathetic system come from both the brain stem and sacral spinal cord. There are no vertebral or paravertebral ganglia in this system, instead the ganglia are found adjacent to the effector organ. These include the otic, sphenopalantine and ciliary ganglia.

43. **DE**
In summarising data for presentation and statistical analysis the arithmetic mean of a population of observations and the standard deviation, which is the mean of the difference of each observation from the mean, may be calculated. It is more usual to quote the standard error of mean (SEM). The mean however should only be calculated for normally distributed observations. If, for example, they show skew distribution, then non-parametric statistics should be used with calculation of the median, the value in the middle of a series of observations arranged in order of size, and the range.

44. AE (APTT ↑)

Heparin, a mixture of sulphated polysaccharides, is an anti-coagulant found in granules of mast cells, wandering cells found in tissues rich in connective tissue. It facilitates the action of anti-thrombin III, a circulating protease inhibitor that binds to thrombin and inhibits it. It exerts its effect by binding to anti-thrombin II and altering its affinity for thrombin. It is not absorbed from gastro-intestinal or sublingual sites. Heparin is metabolised in the liver by an enzyme called heparinase and the metabolic products excreted in the urine.

45. ACE

Thyroxine is one of the hormones produced in the thyroid gland and is chemically a derivative of tyrosine, having four iodine residues attached. The hormone circulates bound to plasma proteins, less than 0.1% of the total circulating hormone being in the free form. Together with the other thyroid hormone, tri-iodothyronine, it plays an important role in the production of heat and in growth. Hypothyroidism in children is associated with retarded bone age in addition to failure of mental and general physical development. Calcitonin is a polypeptide hormone produced by the C cells of the thyroid. It contributes to calcium metabolism, but its role in the human is incompletely defined.

46. ABD

Ether has an MAC of 1.92, enflurane an MAC of 1.68.

47. ABCE

Pancuronium is a biquaternary ammonium structure, highly polar, and does not cross the placenta in significant amounts. Cardio-vascularly, it causes tachycardia, by sympathomimetic and vagolytic mechanisms, accompanied by normotension or slight hypertension. Streptomycin and all aminoglycosides prevent pre junctional release of acetyl choline by blocking calcium ion entry into the neurone.

48. BCE

Cyanide ions are rapidly converted to thiocyanate in the liver, high levels of which cause acute toxic syndromes. This conversion is brought about by rhodanase, a liver enzyme. Patients with vitamin B_{12} deficiency may have their symptoms made worse as nitro-prusside impairs the metabolism of cyanocobalamin. Thiocyanate inhibits both the uptake and binding of iodine.

49. AD
Nitrates are metabolised to nitrites which along with prilocaine can cause methaemoglobinaemia. Methylene blue is used to treat it. Procaine and cinchocaine do not cause it.

50. ABD
Joint pain can also follow chronic use of high inspired oxygen at atmospheric pressure. The damage to the alveoli is thought to be brought about by free radicals. The central nervous system is only damaged by hyperbaric oxygen. The renal and cardiovascular systems are not affected.

51. D
Clonidine is a central post ganglionic α_2 antagonist. Hexamethonium acts as an antagonist at autonomic ganglia, propranolol is a β-antagonist, amyl nitrate a venodilator, and tubocurarine is both a ganglion blocker and releases histamine.

52. CDE
Amiloride is a potassium sparing diuretic, hyperkalaemia can occur. Morphine causes constipation. The megaloblastic anaemia of phenytoin is caused by altered absorption and metabolism of folates. Phenacetin has been implicated in causing renal papillary necrosis, 0.2% of patients receiving isoniazid develop peripheral neuropathy.

53. D α_1 = post synaptic α_2 = presynaptic
Labetalol is a drug with both α and β blocking actions, the β blocking action is more long lasting than the α blocking.

54. AB
Atracurium is broken down by Hoffman degradation at pH 7.4. Suxamethonium is unstable at alkaline pH and should not be mixed with thiopentone. Gallamine forms a stable solution in water unaffected by mixing with thiopentone. The two benzodiazepines are poorly soluble in water and unaffected by pH.
Midazolam becomes lipid soluble c̄ body pH

55. ABC
Aspirin and phenylbutazone displace warfarin from protein binding sites, whereas cimetidine diminishes the activity of mixed function oxidases in the liver thus reducing the metabolism of warfarin. Rifampicin and griseofulvin both induce microsomal enzymes and reduce warfarin levels.

56. DE

Prilocaine is used in the same concentrations as lignocaine, it is very stable in solution, with a longer duration of action than lignocaine. The methaemoglobinaemia is caused by degradation products and it is metabolised in the kidney, lungs, and liver.

57. A

Salbutamol is a β2 agonist and is used to relax the uterus. Receptors in the uterus are stimulatory, thus adrenaline and noradrenaline have an overall stimulatory effect. Acetyl choline is also stimulatory, and there are no dopaminergic receptors in the uterus, but dopamine has a slight α effect.

58. ABCDE

Practolol is β1 selective and has no effect on bronchial smooth muscle. This selectivity gives it a cardiac effect. Side effects include psoriasis, hyperkeratosis, dry eyes, SLE and sclerosing peritonitis.

59. BC

Both promethazine and thiopentone in small doses increase sensitivity to pain, and chlorpromazine has no innate analgesic action. Fentanyl is a potent synthetic opioid, and pentazocine is a partial agonist at both μ and kappa receptors.

60. BDE

Atropine decreases gut motility, and is less sedative and more inhibitory to secretions than hyoscine. The L form is the more active, it crosses the blood brain barrier, and has an excitatory effect centrally, including central vagal stimulation which results in an initial bradycardia.

61. BDE

Their anti emetic action is by antagonising dopamine receptors at the chemoreceptor trigger zone. Central dopamine antagonists can cause dystonia and extra-pyramidal effects. They have no effect on pulse rate and blood pressure. The effects on lower oesophageal tone are local and antagonised by atropine.

62. ADE

Ranitidine is an H_2 antagonist. Gastrin and histamine both increase gastric acid secretion. Sympathetic amines inhibit gastric secretions, and glycopyrrolate is an atropine like drug.

63. AC
The synthesis of adrenaline is:

Tyrosine—›L-Dopa—›Dopamine—›Noradrenaline—›Adrenaline.

64. ABCDE
Hypothermia, hypokalaemia, and aminoglycoside antibiotics all potentiate curare. Ether causes myoneural block which potentiates curare. Pyridostigmine is an anticholinesterase.

65. ABCD
Nitrates cause, venodilatation and venous pooling, decreased cardiac output and myocardial work, increased meningeal blood flow due to loss of arteriolar tone, and lowered pulmonary vascular resistance. They lower the left atrial pressure.

66. CE
Physostigmine, an anticholinesterase, and pilocarpine a muscarinic agonist, are parasympathomimetic reducing pupil size. Trimetaphan is a ganglion blocker, but as the predominant tone in the pupil is parasympathetic, paralysis of both systems at the ganglion results in dilation. Guanethidine is an adrenergic blocking drug and reduces sympathetic tone. Atropine is a muscarinic blocking drug, so unopposed sympathetic tone produces dilatation.

67. BCD
Digoxin is used in the treatment of atrial arrhythmias. Verapamil is used in the treatment of supraventricular tachycardias. Disopyramide is used to maintain sinus rhythm after DC conversion, mexiletine is used as an oral preparation to follow stabilisation of ventricular arrhythmias with lignocaine. Tocainide, is said to have a quinidine like action.

68. ABE
Dantrolene prevents release of Ca^{++} from the sarcoplasmic reticulum. Nifedipine blocks Ca^{++} influx into vascular smooth muscle cells via calcium channels. Digoxin affects Na^+ and K^+ dependent ATPase allowing slow increase in intracellular calcium. Hydralazine acts on cyclic-GMP systems in smooth muscle, and halothane has no effect on Ca^{++} flux.

69. B
Aspirin has its analgesic action via inhibition of prostaglandin synthesis. Fentanyl crosses the dura and enters the CSF, it acts locally at spinal receptors and is also carried caudally to central receptors. Acupuncture and rubbing the injured part work by the same mechanism of preventing onward transmission of nocio-receptor input at the spinal cord level. Epidural bupivicaine has a local anaesthetic action.

70. A
Cocaine produces vasoconstriction by potentiation of noradrenaline at sympathetic nerve terminals. All of the other named agents have no vasoconstrictive action.

71. BCDE
Dextrans are not used for their calorific value, but as plasma expanders. The smaller molecular weight molecules are excreted in the kidney, and also improve the viscosity of the blood. They are polysaccharides produced by the action of bacteria on sucrose. Itching, urticaria and joint pain occur in less than 10%

72. ADE
Halothane has a direct depressant effect on uterine smooth muscle, whereas β-agonists depress via β receptors, and are used to suppress premature labour, a role formerly fulfilled by ethyl alcohol. Ketamine increases sympathetic tone. Neuromuscular blocking drugs have no effect on uterine smooth muscle.

73. AB
Thiopentone is a salt of thiobarbituric acid and in 2.5% solution it has a pH of 10.5. It is metabolised in the liver by oxidation of its side chains, slowly, to inactive metabolites. It is antanalgesic, unstable in solution and is stored in powder form, the solution is in fact stable for two weeks, but is usually discarded after 48 hours.

74. CDE
Increasing the ventilation in normal lungs increases the alveolar partial pressure and thus the blood tension, similarly increasing cardiac output increases the gradient between the alveoli and the blood allowing increased uptake. At altitude the partial pressure is less because the atmospheric pressure is less. Increasing solubility of the agent decreases the ability of the blood tension to rise.

75. AD
Ecothiopate is an anticholinesterase and can prolong the apnoea due to suxamethonium, propanidid potentiates suxamethonium by partly depolarising cell membranes in the end plate area. Gallamine is a nondepolarising muscle relaxant, and slightly larger doses of suxamethonium are required after pretreatment with gallamine to prevent 'sux' pains. Pilocarpine is a muscarinic agonist, skeletal muscle receptors are nicotinic. Monoamine oxidase inhibitors have no effect on skeletal muscle.

76. BCD E
The toxic effect of the aminoglycosides involves the eighth cranial nerve and can affect both vestibular and auditory function, they accumulate in the perilymph. They do not cause optic atrophy, although streptomycin has been implicated in optic nerve dysfunction. They block calcium channels, thus potentiating neuromuscular blockade. Renal function is only mildly impaired in 8–26% of patients, severe acute tubular necrosis occurs rarely.

77. AC E
Absorption from the oral mucosa allows drugs to enter the circulation without first passing through the liver. Food intake slows absorption. In traumatic shock and atropine administration, gastric emptying is delayed, and as the small intestine has the far larger surface area absorption is delayed. Despite the fact that acidic compounds are largely un-ionised in the stomach, the larger surface area of the small intestine and the longer equilibrium time allow greater absorption. [It should still be more Rapid]

78. ACD
Theophylline is a positive inotrope, relaxes bronchial smooth muscle, and acts primarily via phosphodiesterase inhibition although other intracellular mechanisms e.g. effects on calcium availability, and blocking adenosine receptors may also contribute. It causes increased urine flow by decreased absorption of solutes, GFR remains the same. It is a potent CNS stimulant.

79. B
Ketamine is dissolved in water, etomidate in water with propylene glycol. Propanidid was prepared in a 5% solution in polyoxyethylated castor oil. Diazepam is available either in an organic solvent with propylene glycol (Valium) or in an oil/water emulsion (Diazemuls). Althesin was dissolved in Cremophor E L which was implicated in the anaphylactoid reactions which precipitated its withdrawal.

80. ABCDE

Digoxin, morphine, and thiotepa (thiethylperazine) all directly stimulate the chemoreceptor trigger zone. Droperidol, one of the most potent antiemetics, blocks dopamine receptors at the chemoreceptor trigger zone, the same mechanism of action.

PRACTICE EXAM 2

1. BCE

Reduced body sodium as seen in reduction of plasma volume is reflected in reduced sodium flux across the macula densa and increased renin secretion. This leads to increased circulating angiotensin II concentrations which in turn leads to aldosterone release and hence sodium reabsorption. On reduction of blood volume there is reduced venous return and decreased atrial pressure so that vasopressin release is stimulated leading to increased water retention and atrial natriuretic peptide hormone secretion is suppressed, so that sodium retention is again promoted. The fall in arterial pressure in addition also leads to increased sympathetic nerve activity which leads to vasoconstriction, a fall in glomerular capillary pressure and so the glomerular filtration rate is reduced and there is less sodium excretion. The generalised vasoconstriction leads to reduced capillary hydrostatic pressure and hence less fluid is lost to the interstitium. The increased sympathetic nerve activity also promotes renin release.

2. ABCE

Tetany results from hypocalcaemia or alkalaemia. Hypocalcaemia may result from a number of conditions including parathyroidectomy and renal disease. It may also result from malabsorption. In the malabsorption syndrome or gluten sensitivity (coeliac disease) there is a failure to absorb fat. Calcium absorption may also be reduced owing to the formation of insoluble calcium soaps. Alkalaemia may be produced by hyperventilation in which acid is lost in the form of CO_2 or in pyloric stenosis in which acid is lost. In alkalaemia the total calcium content is unchanged, but there is an increase in plasma protein ionization and this 'mops up' calcium.

3. AB

Carrier molecules within the cell membrane are ATPases which catalyse the hydrolysis of ATP which provides energy. The

Na^+-K^+ ATPase also known as the sodium pump uses the energy to extrude three sodium ions and take up two potassium ions into the cell. It is made of two α and two β subunits, each α subunit having a molecular weight of about 95,000 and each β subunit a molecular weight of about 40,000. The subunits have binding sites to which cardiac glycosides, such as ouabaine bind, inhibiting the activity. The normal cell volume and pressure depends on this pump. In its absence, sodium and potassium ions move down concentration gradients and water follows. Generation of an action potential depends on altered ionic conductances of the membrane. The pump is responsible for the ionic distribution across the cell membrane, but the resting permeability to sodium is low so that when a large nerve or muscle is poisoned it runs down slowly and action potentials are not affected for a long time.

4. **BDE**
Haemoglobin is built of 4 subunits. Each consists of a ferrous iron containing haem group attached near the centre of a protein made up of over 140 amino acids. In normal haemoglobin (HbA) the protein chains are two sets of 141 amino acid alpha chains and two 146 amino acid beta chains. Each molecule of haemoglobin combines with 4 moles of oxygen so that when fully saturated each gram of haemoglobin binds 1.39 ml oxygen. The solubility of oxygen of plasma at body temperature is 0.003 ml/100 ml. Dying blood cells are phagocytosed by the macrophages of the mono-nuclearphagocytic system (also called the reticuloendothelial system). Haemoglobin acts as a buffer, binding hydrogen ions, this capacity being greater in reduced haemoglobin.

5. **ABD**
Calcium is present in the plasma in a total concentration of 2.2–2.6 mmol/l and exists in three forms, protein bound, complexed and ionised. Ionised plasma calcium is normally held constant within narrow limits. Low ionised calcium may result from removal of the parathyroid glands or from hyperventilation. A decrease in serum calcium increases the neuromuscular excitability. It also increases the slope of diastolic depolarisation of conducting tissue in the heart so that heart rate is increased. Hypocalcaemia stimulates the release of parathyroid hormone which in turn tends to restore concentrations to normal. Calcitonin secretion is inhibited by low calcium ion concentrations.

6. **ABC**

Excitation arising anywhere in the atria or ventricles spreads out until all the fibres are brought into play, so that, in contrast to skeletal muscle when stimulated responds with excitation of all fibres or shows no response at all – all or none response. Cardiac muscle has a prolonged refractory period which protects the heart from too rapid re-excitation, which could impair its function as a pump. It also prevents recycling of excitation in the muscle network. Heart muscle can contract isometrically and isotonically. In contrast to skeletal muscle, heart muscle derives energy largely from oxidative metabolism. It can also use a number of substrates, including lactic acid and free fatty acids.

7. **B**

The normal arterial PO_2 is approximately 100 mm Hg. Thus the value of 60 mm Hg is very low indicating hypoxaemia. The arterial PCO_2 however is lower than normal indicating that there has been hyperventilation in response to the lowered PaO_2. This hyperventilation would account for the elevation in pH to 7.45. Atelectasis is a condition in which there is a failure of large parts of the lungs to be inflated and results from interference in the production or efficiency of surfactant. In this case there would be elevation of $PaCO_2$ and a reduced PaO_2.

8. **ABE**

The cerebrospinal fluid (c.s.f.) has a number of functions including the provision of a pathway for the removal of products of cerebral metabolism. It is normally clear and colourless. Turbidity commonly due to an increased number of red or white cells, or discolouration resulting from bleeding, are always abnormal. A yellow colour may be due to an elevated plasma bilirubin or to bilirubin formed after subarachnoid haemorrhage. Normal c.s.f. contains no more than 5 lymphocytes/ml. When the pressure is recorded in the lumbar subarachnoid space with the patient in a lateral recumbant position the pressure is normally 4–15 mm Hg.

9. **CD**

Under normal circumstances the PCO_2 is more important in the control of respiration than the PaO_2, the peripheral chemoreceptors not being stimulated until the arterial PaO_2 falls to 60 mm Hg. Increasing ventilation results in a fall in the alveolar CO_2 partial pressure. Oxygen is less affected as inspired oxygen remains constant. However in voluntary hyperpnoea the partial pressure of oxygen may be increased, for example up to 140 mm Hg as compared to a normal value of 100 mm Hg. The difference between mixed venous blood and alveolar gas is much less in the case of CO_2 than in the case of O_2 because of the shallowness of the CO_2 dissociation curve. Thus a ventilation perfusion imbalance has only a small effect on the arterial PCO_2. In the case of oxygen, the relatively oxygen deficient blood from the regions of high perfusion pulls the mean partial pressure of oxygen down to that of mixed venous blood.

10. **DE** *Why not A CDE ? This is what they give in the answer!*
Cardiac output is the product of stroke volume and heart rate. The contractility of the myocardium exerts a major influence on stroke volume. Both noradrenaline and adrenaline increase the contractility of the heart as well as increasing heart rate. Increased sympathetic activity increases cardiac output. In an Olympic class runner cardiac output can increase by 25–30 l/min giving a cardiac output of 30–35 l/min. In non-conditioned adults the maximum increase is about 20 l/min.

11. **ABC**
Renal blood flow is determined using a clearance technique, substituting in the Fick equation the quantity removed [R] by the amount appearing in the urine.

$$\text{Blood flow} = \frac{R}{A\text{-}V} \qquad \text{Renal plasma flow} = \frac{U\,V}{[A]\text{-}[V]}$$

where U = urinary concentration of substance employed, V = volume of urine produced, and [A] and [V] are the concentrations of the substance in the renal artery and vein. Certain substances such as para-amino hippuric acid are virtually completely cleared on their passage through the kidney so that the venous concentration becomes zero. Estimates of renal blood flow give a value of some 1200 ml/min or about 20% of the resting cardiac output. Renal blood flow is autoregulated, remaining remarkably constant at blood pressures between 90 and 200 mm Hg. However renal blood flow may be reduced in situations such as haemorrhage and exercise. Over 90% of the blood passes to the cortex and very little passes to the medulla.

12. **AE**
Calcium absorption takes place largely in the duodenum. It is controlled by the body's needs, being increased when supplies are

low and when requirements are high, as in growing children and lactating women. Calcium is largely absorbed via an active process, but some passive diffusion does occur. The vitamin D metabolite 1,25 dihydroxycholecalciferol increases absorption. It is blocked by oxalates and phosphates which form insoluble salts with calcium ions in the intestinal lumen. Similarly fatty acids form soaps with calcium ions blocking absorption.

13. **ACE**

Following hepatectomy animals survive for only a day or two. There is a fall in blood sugar with accompanying muscle weakness, convulsions and coma. Since the liver is the chief site of deamination of amino acids and the only organ in which urea is formed there is a progressive fall in blood urea and a rise in blood amino acids. Jaundice develops with accumulation of bilirubin in tissues and blood and its excretion in urine. There is reduced coagulation because of a fall in plasma prothrombin and fibrinogen.

14. **BD**

The excretion of acid by the kidney is mainly determined by the diet. Protein diets for example contain large amounts of sulphur which is oxidised to sulphate producing a metabolic acidosis. Hydrogen ions are excreted in various forms including inorganic phosphates, but this does not depend on the plasma inorganic phosphate. About 75% of the non-carbonic acid is excreted in combination with ammonium, synthesised in the renal tubule, mainly through the breakdown of glutamine catalysed by glutaminase. Carbonic anhydrase is required for the effective absorption of bicarbonate and for every bicarbonate ion absorbed, a hydrogen ion is excreted into the tubule. Even though hydrogen ions secreted into the tubule are not excreted as such, overall the hydrogen ion excretion is still affected. Aldosterone also promotes excretion of hydrogen and ammonium ions, but does not control it.

15. **BCE**

Hypovolaemia results in a decrease in afferent impulses from the volume receptors which leads to an increase in plasma vasopressin concentrations and a fall in urine flow. Glomerular filtration rate also decreases with volume depletion and hence the amount of sodium filtered and reabsorbed. As a result of the fall of total body sodium there is increased renin release. This in turn leads to increased production of angiotensin II and aldosterone secretion. This hormone then promotes the retention of sodium.

16. ADE

During pregnancy there is an increased demand for blood supply by the uterus and other organs such as the kidney. This is met by an increased cardiac output and blood volume. Blood volume increases as a result of rises in both plasma and erythrocyte volumes, but the former is greater so that there is a decrease in packed cell volume. This is especially noticeable in pre-eclampsia. Plasma iron levels fall, but there is increased iron binding capacity. Plasma albumin concentrations fall but globulin concentrations and those of fibrinogen increase.

17. BC

Characteristically physiological responses such as those involving enzymes are slowed on cooling. Thus in muscle contraction there is a slower rate of interaction between actin and myosin and a reduced rate of re-uptake of calcium by the sarcoplasmic reticulum, so that there is a slower rate of relaxation. A slower conduction velocity in the nerve and muscle fibres would lengthen the latency between the onset of contraction and the stimulus, but would not affect the actual time course of the mechanical response. Muscle contraction can still occur on arrest of the circulation or in an isolated muscle and this response is temperature sensitive.

18. ABCDE

The lumbar and sacral nerves have long spinal roots that descend in the dural sac to reach their appropriate vertebral level of exit. These roots are called cauda equinae as they have the appearance of a horse's tail. A lesion in this region results in pain and asymmetric motor and sensory involvement of multiple roots, it may also result in an autonomous bladder, loss of voluntary control, loss of anal reflex and a large residual urine. There may also be evidence of autonomic disturbances.

19. ACE

The values cited are those for an adult. Pulmonary ventilation is the respiratory rate times tidal volume and in this case is 7.5 l/min. Because of the dead space alveolar ventilation is less than pulmonary ventilation. The latter may be derived from the equation alveolar ventilation = respiratory rate x (tidal volume – dead space) and in this case is 6 l/min. The ventilation: perfusion ratio is the alveolar ventilation divided by the cardiac output, namely 0.86.

20. CE

The glomerular filtrate and interstitial fluid are formed by filtration across the capillary. It occurs as a result of a balance of forces – the hydrostatic pressure forcing fluid out of the capillary and the plasma oncotic pressure tending to draw it into the capillary. In salivary secretion, the primary secretion resembles an ultrafiltrate, but is the product of active transport and contains amylase. Bile is concentrated by rapid reabsorption of water and electrolytes. Sweat production is from the exocrine sweat glands, which are widely distributed over the surface of the body.

21. CD

With a heart rate of 80 the duration of the cardiac cycle, namely the interval between each QRS complex is 0.75 sec. The P-R interval during which atrial depolarisation and conduction through the A-V node occurs is on average 0.18 sec (range 0.12–0.2). The QRS interval during which ventricular depolarisation occurs is of 0.08–0.10/sec duration. The S-T interval corresponding to ventricular depolarisation is 0.32 sec. Protodiastole, which is the period when the ventricular muscle is fully contracted and the already falling pressure drops most rapidly, lasts about 0.04 sec and ends with the aortic and pulmonary valves producing the second heart sound.

22. ACE

Exposure to hyperbaric oxygen produces increases in the oxygen dissolved in the blood, but not the maximum amount of oxygen carried by the haemoglobin. Cardiac output decreases as a result of increased vagal tone and there is decreased blood flow through the brain and kidney. While hyperbaric oxygen is of therapeutic value, the use of 100% oxygen at elevated pressure accelerates the onset of oxygen toxicity. An elevation of PO_2 in the cells affects the activity of many enzymes in tissue metabolism so that, for example, oxidation of glucose and pyruvic acid is inhibited. Typical symptoms evoked by hyperbaric oxygen are tracheobronchial irritation, dizziness, nausea, ringing in the ears and eventually convulsions and coma. At 6 atmospheres convulsions develop within a few minutes.

23. ABCDE

The hypothalamus sits at the gateway to the brain, monitoring electrical information from the limbic system and brain stem and transducing it into nervous and humoral stimuli, including the output of vasopressin involved in water balance. The hypothalamus also directly participates in many motivational behaviours such as eating, drinking and sexual behaviour, as well as certain vegetative functions such as temperature regulation. In addition, it controls the autonomic nervous system and hence influences blood pressure.

24. CD
Vitamin B_{12} is necessary for red blood cell formation because of its ability to make another B vitamin, folic acid, available for use by bone marrow. Deficiency leads to pernicious anaemia. In anaemias of this type the red cells, although they are fewer, are larger than normal; it is thus a macrocytic anaemia. The oxygen capacity of blood is approximately 1.39 g O_2/g haemoglobin. Thus 110 g/l would carry about 150 ml O_2/l blood.

25. BCE
The placenta is the fetal lung and about 53% of the fetal cardiac output goes through the placenta. It returns to the fetus via the umbilical vein, enters the right atrium and passes through the foramen ovale to the left atrium. Blood does pass to the pulmonary artery, but because the pressure in the pulmonary artery is higher than in the aorta, blood passes through the ductus arteriosus to the aorta. Thus relatively unsaturated blood from the right ventricles is diverted to the trunk and lower body. At birth the lungs are inflated and there is a fall in pulmonary resistance to blood flow so pulmonary artery pressure falls. The pressure in the right atrium falls below that in the left atrium, so the flap-like valve closes over the foramen ovale. The ductus arteriosus begins to constrict shortly after birth due to the release of prostaglandins, so that the patency of this vessel can be maintained with aspirin.

26. ABCD
In contrast to compliance of the lungs and thorax combined, lung compliance, a static measurement, is derived in practice from a plot of volume/transpulmonary pressure relationships, measured during the brief periods of no flow when the subject takes a brief breath incrementally. The subject inspires from a spirometer making stepwise increases in the lung volume pausing after each step to allow measurement of the pressure and volume. The glottis remains open so that the alveolar pressure equals atmospheric pressure. The transpulmonary pressure is given by the intrapulmonary pressure minus the intrapleural pressure. Direct measurement of intra-pulmonary pressure is not normally possible, but a close approximation can be obtained by measuring the pressure in the oesophagus. The oesophagus being flaccid, the pressure can be

measured in the thoracic segment of the oesophagus. The lung compliance is approximately 0.2 l/cm H_2O.

27. BD

Of all the tissues listed, heart muscle has the greatest A-V oxygen difference of approximately 114 ml/l. It has a very high flow rate of 84.0 ml/100 g tissue, but a very high oxygen consumption of 97 ml/100 g/min. At the other extreme the kidneys have a low A-V difference of 14 ml/l. This results from a high flow rate of 420.0 ml/100 g/min despite the relatively high oxygen consumption of 6.0 ml/100 g/min. The A-V difference across the brain is also relatively high as is that for skeletal muscle. The latter has a relatively low oxygen consumption, but a very low flow rate of 2.7 ml/100 g/min. The skin also has a relatively low A-V difference.

28. ACD

The resting membrane potential depends on the unequal distribution of ions across the cell membrane and the permeability of the membrane. If the membrane potential depended solely on potassium ions the membrane potential would be given by the equation

$$\text{Potential} = 60 \log x \, [K^+]_{out} \big/ [K^+]_{in}$$

with a potassium ratio of 1:30 this is -90 mV. Direct measurement shows the membrane potential to be about -70 to -80 mV. The ionic distribution depends on a sodium pump and so there is a decrease in prolonged exposure to anoxia. The rate of conductance of an action potential depends on the diameter of the fibre, but not the resting membrane potential.

29. BC

The carotid bodies lie above and near the bifurcation of the common carotid artery on both sides of the neck and are supplied by the carotid sinus nerve which travels in the glossopharyngeal nerve. Together with the aortic bodies they form the peripheral chemoreceptors responding to changes in oxygen, carbon dioxide and hydrogen ion concentrations in the blood. They are largely sensitive to the partial pressure of oxygen and are thus stimulated on reduced blood flow which contributes to the increased chemoreceptor discharge on haemorrhage. The central chemoreceptors sensitive to changes in pH and hence CO_2, are located in the medulla on the ventral surface of the brain stem.

30. CD

If hypotonic urine is being produced, then there is reduced water reabsorption. This results from reduced permeability of the collecting duct to water so that water cannot move down the concentration gradient. Such a low permeability of the collecting duct to water is seen in the presence of low concentrations or absence of vasopressin. Since urine on filtration and in the proximal tubule is isotonic to plasma, the production of a hypotonic urine means that sodium ions may have been actively absorbed. Production of a hypotonic urine is unrelated to glomerular filtration rate.

31. DE

The most common cause of oversecretion of thyroid hormone is Graves' disease, though TSH secreting tumours have been reported. Hyperthyroidism is characterised by increased metabolic rate and weight loss. There is negative nitrogen balance resulting from inhibition of protein synthesis and/or stimulation of protein breakdown with increased nitrogen excretion. There is also nervousness, increased pulse pressure, fine tremor of outstretched fingers and heat intolerance with associated warm skin and sweating.

32. ABE

The cerebellum is intimately associated with all aspects of motor control. Its function relates to the control of the timing, duration and strength of a movement. Thus a lesion in the vestibulocerebellum results in a loss of equilibrium and an ataxic gait. A neocerebellar lesion is associated with decomposition of movement, dysmetria or the inability to stop a movement at the appropriate time, intention tremor and adiadochokinesia or the inability to make rapidly alternating movements. No spontaneous movements are associated with cerebellar disease. Muscle weakness is associated with lesions in the tracts from the cerebral cortex.

33. BDE

In Europe the onset of puberty has been declining at the rate of 1–3 months per decade for more than 175 years. It is characterised by activation of the gonads by gonadotrophins, the release of which are stimulated by pulsatile release of GnRH. Although puberty is the time when gonadal development is such that reproduction is possible, ova do not start to form in the ovary, as they are present in the ovary at birth. Another feature is the increased secretion of adrenal androgens. Early, but otherwise normal, pubertal patterns of gonadotrophin secretion from the pituitary are described as precocious puberty. Among the commonest causes are lesions of the hypothalamus.

34. ABE

The main signs of right ventricular failure are found in the systemic venous system. Thus the increased venous pressure causes distension of veins above the clavicles. There is a large systolic venous wave which can be seen in the neck and felt over the liver which is also enlarged. There is dependent oedema. The extravascular loss of sodium and water results in increased aldosterone production.

35. ACDE

The rate of airflow is directly proportional to the driving pressure which is directly related to the alveolar pressure and indirectly proportional to the airway resistance. This is given by the equation

Airflow = Alveolar pressure/Airway resistance

Airway resistance depends on bronchomotor tone and the transmural pressures of the airway. The bronchiolar tone depends on humoral factors such as histamine and the autonomic nerves, both sympathetic and parasympathetic. Dynamic airway collapse would not be seen during quiet breathing as it only occurs during marked expiratory effects.

36. ABCE

Hyponatraemia is associated with Addison's disease, a condition in which there is underproduction of the adrenocortical hormones and which is dominated by a lack of mineralocorticoids. Hyponatraemia is also characteristic of the syndrome of inappropriate vasopressin secretion, so called as the vasopressin concentrations are inappropriately high for the concurrent plasma osmolality. Plasma osmolality may be elevated by non-osmotic stimulation of vasopressin release acutely, as for example during surgery, or chronically as in respiratory disease, by drugs or in ectopic secretion from tumours. Despite the water retention and fall in plasma osmolality, concentrated urine continues to be excreted. The plasma osmolality may fall so low that water intoxication is seen.

37. BDE

The cells or origin of the vagus, the tenth cranial nerve, lie in the medulla – the nucleus ambiguus. The vagal outflow is blocked by atropine which acts at the postsynaptic receptor. Thus a muscarinic receptor is involved. The effect of vagal stimulation is to slow heart rate. This is achieved through an effect on the S-A node where conductance is increased. Vagal stimulation also produces a fall in the conduction velocity in the A-V node and a reduction in the contractility of the atria.

$Conductance = \dfrac{1}{Resistance}$

38. ABC

The condition originally described would appear to be due to elevated plasma aldosterone. Aldosterone promotes renal excretion of potassium and absorption of osmotically active material, sodium and chloride. The enhanced renal reabsorption of sodium is accompanied by increased reabsorption of water, increased extracellular fluid volume and dilution of colloid and oedema. Fluid loss from the capillaries is also enhaced by reduced plasma oncotic pressure. A decreased secretion of vasopressin would cause dehydration not oedema and would not reduce the sodium excretion.

39. AC

Pulse pressure is increased by an increase in stroke volume which varies arterial uptake. Increased elastance or decreased compliance also increases pulse pressure. In contrast if stroke volume is held constant pulse pressure is reduced by increases in heart rate and peripheral resistance. In both cases arterial volume increases with the result that pulse pressure decreases.

40. ABD

On instilling dilute acid into the duodenum, secretin, a polypeptide hormone is released from the mucosa. This hormone stimulates a high output of fluid and bicarbonate from the pancreas and a similar increase in the volume and bicarbonate content of bile. The effects of secretin on the stomach are to reduce gastric motility and inhibit gastric acid production.

41. ABCD

Insulin is produced in the cells of the islets of Langerhans. Immunocytochemically the cells have been shown to contain glucagon. Insulin is a polypeptide with a molecular weight of 6,000 and consists of two chains, A and B, which are linked by two disulphide bonds. A third bond links the two cysteine residues within the A chain. Insulin is a hormone of times of plenty, promoting the uptake of glucose into cells and the conversion to glycogen and triglycerides. Insulin stimulates the uptake of amino acids and in this way could stimulate protein synthesis by providing the precursor amino acid requirements. Insulin has a relatively short half time in plasma of about 10 min.

42. BCD

A solution of 0.9% sodium chloride contains 0.15 M NaCl and has an osmolality of 300 mOsm/kg and is slightly hypertonic to normal human plasma. If 0.9% NaCl is used to perfuse an isolated heart in vitro rhythmicity disappears and the heart stops beating. If calcium ions are added, the heart beats for a while and stops in systole. If potassium ions are added it stops in diastole. If all three ions are present beating continues indefinitely. Ammonium chloride is used to treat metabolic acidosis resulting from vomiting and loss of HCl but can precipitate hepatic coma.

43. ABD

Very little absorption occurs in the stomach, the only substances being absorbed to any appreciable extent are lipid soluble substances as for example ethanol. This includes unionised forms of many weak acids such as triglycerides of acetic and butyric acids. Aspirin or salicylic acid at gastric pH is unionised and fat soluble and hence readily absorbed.

$A^- + H^+ \longleftrightarrow AH$ ie unionised = undissociated!

44. BC

Cortisol is a glucocorticoid and increases the concentration of glucose in the blood by stimulating gluconeogenesis in the liver and to a lesser extent the utilisation of glucose in other tissues. The metabolic effects of cortisol vary with the target tissue. In adipose, muscle and lymphoid tissue it is catabolic, but in the liver it stimulates the synthesis and storage of glycogen. In addition to its effects on metabolism, cortisol acts on the body's defence mechanisms. It leads to reduction in the size of the lymph nodes, involution of the thymus and reduces the number of lymphocytes in the blood. It also contributes to the control of ACTH release, decreasing the concentrations of the trophic hormones via negative feedback.

45. ABE

If a population of values shows a normal or Gaussian distribution, then a plot of the frequency of any given value against the values has a bell-like curve, with the mean, median and mode corresponding to the peak. If values show such a distribution, then parametric statistics may be used. It can be shown that 63.27% of the observations lie within one standard deviation and 95.45% within two. The standard error of mean (SEM) for large populations is given by SD/n and that for small populations by SD/n-1. The coefficient of variation is given by SD/mean x 100%.

46. ABE

Beclomethasone is given as an inhaler in asthma and this can result in oral candidiasis, in sufficient doses adrenal suppression can occur. It suppresses cortisol excretion because it is a synthetic glucocorticoid.

47. ABE

Atropine crosses into the brain and causes excitation, it also causes bradycardia in low doses due to central vagal stimulation, the smooth muscle of the bronchi relax due to unopposed sympathetic action. Its action on the stomach is to lower tone and activity, its cardiac effect is to block vagal effects at the SA node.

48. B

The major pathway of metabolism is via conjugation with glucuronide.

49. CE

The respiratory depressant effect of fentanyl is due to a direct effect on the respiratory centre, and is reversed by naloxone as is the analgesia. Recirculation in the bile can result in late respiratory depression. Pentazocine is an agonist/antagonist and will reduce the action of fentanyl. Opiates are additive.

50. BC

Nitrous oxide is produced by the reaction:

$$NH_4 \longrightarrow 2H_2O + N_2O$$

The principal impurities are due to overheating and are nitric oxide and nitrogen dioxide. Thymol is a preservative added to halothane, and phosgene is a breakdown product of chloroform.

51. BDE

Hypokalaemia is associated with sensitivity to curare. Neomycin produces neuromuscular block by inhibiting acetylcholine release presynaptically, the block is also potentiated by excess magnesium ions which reduce the release of acetylcholine. The effect of temperature is to reduce the block between 37°C and 30–34°C below which it is potentiated. Physostigmine is an anticholinesterase.

52. ABD

β-blockers reduce systolic and diastolic blood pressure and cardiac output. They are used in the treatment of angina, and must be used with caution in diabetics because of their metabolic effects. Phenylepherine is a sympathomimetic amine and thus is antagonised by β-blockers.

53. **BCDE**
A 2.5% solution of thiopentone has a pH of 10.8. About 70% of thiopentone is protein bound, and at physiological pH it exists as ionised and unionised species. It is metabolised slowly, 10–15% of the drug in the body is metabolised per hour. In subanaesthetic doses it is anti-analgesic.

54. **AD**
Dextrans are formed by the action of bacteria on sucrose. High molecular weight dextrans are not deleterious to renal function, but low molecular weight dextrans improve microcirculation. They are slowly oxidised in the liver over a number of weeks, and have a very long half life in excess of three days.

55. **AC**
Procaine has a short duration of action because its ester linkage is rapidly hydrolysed by plasma esterases, it has no effect on vascular tone. It has a pKa of 9, so is 90–95% ionised at pH 7.4. It is rapidly hydrolysed, so is not excreted unchanged in the urine, however it forms salts with penicillin and thus prolongs its action by limiting absorption.

56. **ABDE**
Penicillin is the drug of choice in meningococcal meningitis. Flucloxacillin is penicillinase resistant, staphylococci produce penicillinase. Aminoglycosides cause mild renal tubular impairment in 8–26% of patients. Although co-trimoxazole is largely bacteriostatic it is actually bactericidal in some organisms. Chloramphenicol is the mainstay of the treatment of typhoid.

57. **A**
The transmitter at autonomic ganglia is acetylcholine, the receptors are nicotinic.

58. **BCD**   *What about delayed stomach emptying in atropine?*
Particulate antacids may stimulate secretions into the stomach. Gastric secretions are reduced by metoclopramide which encourages peristalsis into the duodenum, by cimetidine which is an H_2 antagonist, and atropine which is a muscarinic antagonist. Pyridostigmine is an anticholinesterase resulting in muscarinic stimulation of gastric secretions.

59. ACD
Dopamine is produced in vivo by the action of dopa decarboxylase on L-dopa. If given systemically it does not pass the blood brain barrier, and although it is a transmitter at the chemoreceptor trigger zone, it does not therefore cause nausea. It is chronotropic and inotropic and can cause tachyarrhythmias, and is a pressor agent.

60. AE
Digoxin increases intracellular calcium, and nifedipine blocks calcium channels. Hydralazine activates cyclic GMP, phentolamine is an α-blocker, and diazoxide relaxes vascular smooth muscle directly.

61. CD
Ecothiopate is an anticholinesterase which constricts the pupil. Pilocarpine is a muscarinic agonist which constricts the pupil. Homatropine as a muscarinic antagonist and adrenaline as a sympathetic agonist both dilate the pupil. Cyanide causes a transient stimulation of the CNS before respiratory arrest occurs, but has no specific action on the pupil.

62. ABCE
Both lignocaine and phenytoin are useful, and propranolol may also have a role, but it often causes other dysrhythmias. Calcium salts may aggravate the dysrhythmias. Potassium decreases the binding of digoxin to the heart.

63. A
In competitive antagonism, the antagonist combines with the same receptors as the agonist, but without pharmacological effect, the log dose response curve is displaced to the right in a parallel manner, although the maximal response obtained is unaffected. In non-competitive antagonism the slope of the dose-response curve is flattened. The effects are not necessarily equal and opposite.

64. BCDE
Warfarin has its action by reducing liver synthesis of clotting factors, and only achieves its full effect when synthesis is fully suppressed. Vitamin K reverses its effect because it is required to convert pro-factors to active coagulation proteins. Phenylbutazone and barbiturates increase the effect of warfarin by displacement of the warfarin from protein binding sites.

E false → P uso reduction !

65. E

Frusemide is a loop diuretic. It reduces extracellular volume rather than blood volume, and has no effect on blood sugar. It reduces urate excretion and hyperuricaemia is common. Its intrarenal mechanism is to inhibit reabsorption of electrolytes in the ascending loop of Henle. Potassium is lost in the distal tubule and hypokalaemia can result.

66. BCE

Commercial heparin is prepared from bovine lung and porcine intestinal mucosa. It is present in mast cells in the form of big heparin, from which it is released in anaphylactic shock when it is rapidly ingested and destroyed by macrophages. Its physiological function in this situation is unknown. It is an antithrombin and releases and ~~stablises~~ enzymes which are lipid hydrolysing.

stimulates

67. ABCE

Metoclopramide has a central anti-emetic effect as well as its peripheral effects. Domperidone, cyclizine, and hyoscine are all used in motion sickness. Imipramine has no action against motion sickness.

68. BCE

Both glibenclamide and β-blockers lower blood sugar. All thiazides are capable of causing hyperglycaemia, and adrenaline raises blood sugar by its β action on the islet cells.

69. ABC

Isoprenaline is a β-agonist, aminophylline acts by increasing intracellular cyclic AMP, the second messenger of the sympathetic receptor. Mephentermine is a direct and indirect sympathomimetic amine. Methoxamine acts on peripheral α-receptors and has virtually no action on the heart, labetalol is an α and β blocker.

70. ABC

Monoamine oxidase inhibitors lead to the accumulation of 5-hydroxytryptamine, dopamine and noradrenaline within the neurone. Pethidine, tricyclic antidepressants and sympathomimetic amines can all interact and hypertensive crisis can result. There is no interaction with curare or halothane.

71. E

Morphine commonly causes the release of histamine. Chlorpheniramine and promethazine are antihistaminic drugs.

118

72. ABDE

It is suggested that a least two doses of lithium be omitted before anaesthesia. Trimetaphan is primarily a ganglion blocker but also has some neuromuscular blocking action of its own, diazepam seems to potentiate neuromuscular block, and ether produces some neostigmine reversible neuromuscular block, as well as generally depressing neuronal conduction. Suxamethonium and competitive blockers do not potentiate each other in doses below that which produces dual block.

73. BDE

Cinchocaine is a quinoline derivative, 15 times as potent as procaine, and is an amide local anaesthetic, thus it is stable during autoclaving. It has been widely used in spinal anaesthesia. It is also known as dibucaine.

74. BCD

Opioid receptors are distributed throughout the brain and spinal cord. Morphine acts principally at the mu receptor, now divided into two subsets mu_1 and mu_2. Kappa receptors are found in the spinal cord and supraspinally in the cortex, the agonists at these receptors often produce dysphoria. β endorphins are natural agonists at both mu and sigma receptors. Naloxone antagonises at all opioid receptors.

75. ABCDE

Noradrenaline and acetylcholine are present at all levels, 5-hydroxy-tryptamine is present in the mid brain and pons. GABA and glycine are present in spinal and supraspinal interneurones.

76. ABCE

Metabolic acidosis, coma, convulsions, and rarely thrombo-cytopenic purpura, all occur, pulmonary oedema is a late and usually premortem sign. Jaundice does not occur.

77. ~~AE~~ *ACE*

Morphine has a significant but variable first pass metabolism, and aspirin, acetylsalicylic acid is rapidly metabolised at first pass to its active form salicylic acid. ~~Lignocaine and~~ warfarin ~~are both~~ metabolised in the liver but first pass metabolism is not significant. Buprenorphine is excreted largely unchanged in the faeces.

78. CDE

Ketamine produces sympathetic stimulation with tachycardia and a rise in systolic blood pressure. It increases intracranial and intra-ocular pressure. Hallucinations are a characteristic of the emergence delirium associated with ketamine. Muscle tone increases especially in the jaw, and abnormal movements may occur during induction.

79. ABC
The MAC of halothane is highest in infants under six months (1.08%), whereas in the elderly it is 0.64%. Opiates and inhalational agents have additive effects reducing MAC. The antiarrhythmic agents verapamil and nifedipine have no effect on MAC.

80. ABCE
Atracurium is metabolised by spontaneous Hoffman degradation at pH 7.4 and by ester hydrolysis. Metabolism of all drugs is slowed by hypothermia. Laudenasine is one of the non active metabolites of atracurium which in very large doses in animals has a strychnine like analeptic activity, which is not significant in clinical usage. Its speed of onset is slower than suxamethonium at all dosages. In acid pH the molecule is more stable.

PRACTICE EXAM 3

1. ABDE
Haemoglobin is a protein made of 4 subunits, each one containing one atom of ferrous iron. Each iron atom can bind irreversibly to oxygen. Once the haemoglobin has taken up one molecule of oxygen, uptake of additional oxygen is favoured so that the curve relating the percentage saturation of haemoglobin to the PO_2, the oxygen dissociation curve, is sigmoid in nature. If this curve is shifted to the right there is effectively an increase in the P50 which is normally 27 mm Hg in arterial blood. This shift may be produced by an increase in the PCO_2, the temperature, the hydrogen ion concentration and organic phosphates such as ATP and 2,3 diphosphoglycerate. The Bohr effect is the increase in P50 caused by the reaction of haemoglobin with CO_2. On ascent to altitude hyperventilation occurs so that alkalosis occurs which would tend to decrease the P50.

+E ? Ganong p 610
ascent to high altitude : 2,3 DPG ↑ → P50 ↑
See also answer 15

2. **ABE**
   Cardiac muscle has the inherent property of rhythmicity, a property developed to the greatest extent in the S-A node, the so-called pacemaker. The fibres of the cardiac muscle cells form a network or sheet of muscle in which it is difficult to distinguish individual cells and the whole behaves like a syncitium. The cardiac action potential lasts nearly as long as the mechanical events, so that the heart muscle is refractory for extended periods and cannot go into a sustained contraction or tetanus.

3. **C**
   The pH of 7.43 is the alkaline side of the normal pH of 7.4. This does not result from a respiratory disturbance as the elevated PCO_2 of 6.4 kPa would produce an acidosis. It seems to stem from the elevated plasma bicarbonate of 43 mmol/l, the normal value being 24 mmol/l. The elevated pH would suppress respiration bringing the ratio of HCO_3/CO_2 back to normal. Hence as predicted by the Henderson Hasselbach equation

$$pH = 6.1 \log \left(\frac{HCO_3}{0.03 \ PCO_2} \right) - pH \text{ is restored.}$$

4. **B**
   When a limb is immersed in warm water for a period there is an increased oral temperature closely connected with the temperature in the subclavian artery, but no change in the rectal temperature. The rectal temperature reflects deep body temperature which is maintained through a number of mechanisms including vasodilatation. It would require a local fall in the partial pressure of oxygen or a rise in that of carbon dioxide to cause vasodilatation in one arm.

5. **ACDE**
   The stomach plays a role in digestion, salivary amylase being active in the hydrolysis of starch. Protein digestion is minimal, although pepsin does destroy cellular integrity and reduce meat particles. These actions however are not essential for the digestive process. Conditions in the stomach are favourable for the reduction of iron to the ferrous form which is more readily absorbed. Iron deficiency anaemia may thus occur on gastrectomy. Vitamin B_{12} absorption is also impaired as it requires intrinsic factor which is produced in the parietal cells of the gastric mucosa. Duodenal mucosa is leaky and osmotic equilibrium is rapidly achieved so that haemodilution will occur after drinking water.

6. **BDE**
   The decrease in blood volume on haemorrhage produces a drop in the blood pressure which initiates baroreceptor reflexes which restore the pressure towards normal. There is an increased heart rate, but because there is a large drop in stroke volume, cardiac output is not restored to pre-haemorrhage levels. Also important in restoring blood pressure is the increase in total peripheral resistance resulting from increased sympathetic outflow in many peripheral beds, but not those of the heart and brain. There is also an increase in venous tone and reduced venous capacitance. Another important compensatory mechanism, namely reduced formation of tissue fluid, results from the reduced capillary hydrostatic pressure.

7. **DE**
   The functional residual capacity is the volume of air in the lungs at the end of quiet expiration and is a measure of the resting expiratory position. This volume which increases on standing is 3 l and comprises the expiratory reserve volume and the residual volume. The expiratory reserve volume can be measured using a spirometer, but the residual volume is generally measured by introducing a gas into the lungs, allowing it to mix with the air there and then measuring its dilution. The closing volume is that portion of the vital capacity remaining in the lungs when airway closure begins. This occurs as the residual volume is approached in healthy young people.

8. **ACE** *why not D as well?*
   Regulation of temperature is important as a rise in the temperature of the blood flowing to the brain results in confusion and delirium. Temperature is regulated by a balance between heat generation and loss. There are peripheral thermoreceptors in the skin which convey information to the brain via the lateral spinothalamic tract. Thermoreceptors are also found in the central nervous system, in the hypothalamus where thermoregulatory responses are integrated. Heat is lost via a number of mechanisms including vasodilation and sweating, the latter sometimes occurring at the expense of fluid balance.

9. **D**
   On forced expiration the pleural pressure becomes positive, but still is less than that in the alveoli. Pressure in the airways decreases from alveolar to atmospheric along the lung. At some point the pleural pressure will equal the pressure inside the airways and beyond this point the airways are narrowed because of the pressure

gradient across the wall. The narrowing limits the maximal expiratory flow rate.

10. **ABE**

Approximately 80% of the water filtered at the glomerulus is reabsorbed by the time the filtrate has traversed the proximal tubule. This contributes to the increased concentration of PAH and urea and the increased osmotic pressure. Furthermore PAH is secreted into the proximal tubule increasing the concentration further. During a systemic acidosis ammonia is produced by cells of the proximal as well as the distal convoluted tubule.
⌐, it is isotonic at end of prox. tubule

11. **BDE**

Hypothyroidism is generally called myxoedema, which describes the thickening of the skin caused by an increase in the connective tissue with retention of water and mucoproteins. Basal metabolic rate falls; there is a reduced oral temperature and cold is poorly tolerated. The voice is husky and slow. Mental processes are poor and there is a tendency to fall asleep. The hair is coarse and sparse and the skin is dry.

12. **ABCD**

By the fourth week of pregnancy the placenta has developed to such an extent that substances can pass across it from the maternal to the fetal circulation and vice versa. Passage of substances into the fetal circulation is largely related to the molecular weight. Substances with a molecular weight of 1,000 usually cross the placenta by simple diffusion. Fetal fat crosses in two ways, by transfer of fatty acids and cholesterol across the placenta and by synthesis of fat from carbohydrate. Antibodies which are globulins of molecular weight exceeding 100,000 can certainly cross the placenta. Nearly all drugs are of low molecular weight so it is to be expected that the majority can cross the placenta given the appropriate physico-chemical properties.

13. **AE**

When a sound reaches the ear it causes vibrations of the tympanic membrane, which are transmitted via the ossicles in the middle ear to the oval window of the inner ear. The sound energy is transmitted to the perilymph in the inner ear and therefore some structure must permit pressure equilibration. This structure is the oval window which moves out as the stapes moves in. The vibrations of the fluid in the inner ear are converted to nerve impulses, a process involving movement of the basilar membrane. The region of vibration is related to the pitch and the extent of vibration to intensity. There is a power function relationship between the increase in sound pressure and the perceived increase in loudness. Interpretation of the information takes place in the auditory cortex.

14. **BCDE**
The oedema of cirrhosis is localised in the abdominal cavity (ascites). Degeneration of parenchymal cells results in impairment of circulation through the liver and hence hypertension which enhances exudation of fluid into the abdomen. Impaired liver function also results in reduced plasma protein synthesis and hypoalbuminaemia which also contributes to the effective outgoing gradient for filtration of fluid. There is reduced renal clearance of hormones so that aldosterone concentrations are elevated leading to salt and water retention. *inactivation in liver (glucuronide) in*
In unival people hyperaldosteron sun does not produce oedema!

15. **AE** *(hairy)*
The slope and position of the dissociation curve are subject to modification by a number of factors. A shift in the haemoglobin dissociation curve occurs primarily in the region of partial saturation of haemoglobin with oxygen, namely in the region 10–90% saturation. Thus the shift has little significance in the lungs, but is important in the tissues. The curve is shifted in exercise with a fall not only in pH, but with an increase in 2,3 diphosphoglycerate as seen at altitude, thus unloading oxygen when required. In carbon monoxide poisoning the 2,3 diphosphoglycerate is reduced and the curve is shifted to the left.

16. **C**
Alterations in the lung volume are the most significant factors influencing pulmonary vascular resistance. Marked increases or decreases in lung volume cause vascular compression producing an increased vascular resistance. Increased resistance is also seen at altitude because of the hypoxic vasoconstriction. Pulmonary vasoconstriction in response to hypoxia can lead to right ventricular hypertrophy. Vascular resistance however falls in exercise because of the increased recruitment of vascular beds.

17. **BCDE**
Activity of the heart and oxygen consumption would be increased by an increase in heart rate produced by a pacemaker or sympathetic stimulation. A similar effect would be produced by an increase in systemic blood pressure or, by the Laplace relationship, the size of the heart. Parasympathetic stimulation would lead to

reduced heart rate which would reduce oxygen consumption of the myocardial muscle.

18. ACE
The chief muscles of respiration are the diaphragm, supplied by the phrenic nerves which arise in the neck from the cervical roots C3, 4 and 5 and the intercostal muscles supplied by the thoracic inter-costal nerves. These are the inspiratory muscles and when they contract the volume of the thoracic cavity and therefore the lungs is increased. Inspiration is an active process involving muscular activity. Expiration is brought about by the elastic recoil of the lungs. Forced expiration may be brought about by activation of the expiratory muscles such as those of the abdomen.

19. BDE
The filtration fraction is given by the ratio GFR/renal plasma flow. The net driving force for water and solute transport across the glomerulus is a function of two variables - the hydrostatic pressure gradients driving fluid out of the glomerular capillary and into Bowman's capsule and the colloid osmotic pressure bringing fluid into the glomerular capillary. Thus decreasing arterial colloid osmotic pressure results in an increased filtration fraction. When the efferent arterial resistance increases the glomerular filtration rate increases and renal plasma flow decreases resulting in an increase in the filtration fraction. The other factors given all decrease GFR and hence the filtration fraction.

20. CD
Although calcium absorption from the gut is active, it is far from complete. Protein digestion and absorption is a highly efficient process; only 2–5% of ingested protein remaining in the small intestine. The majority of protein is broken down to amino acids which are actively absorbed via a carrier mechanism. Di- and tripeptides are absorbed via a separate mechanism. The small intestine in the fetus and neonate has the capacity to absorb intact polypeptides and proteins and intact protein absorption can also occur in the adult. Following the uptake of the products of fat digestion into the intestinal epithelial cells, long chain fatty acids are re-synthesised into triglycerides with glycerol. Some water is reabsorbed in the colon, but the majority is taken up in the small intestine.

21. AB
In an attack of acute glaucoma the iridocorneal angle becomes

blocked, intraocular pressure rises sharply and blood flow through the retina is impaired. As a consequence of the reduced blood flow the retina can suffer temporary or permanent damage with blindness. The intraocular pressure is considered to be pathologically high when it is about 25 mm Hg in repeated measurements. In an attack of acute glaucoma it can exceed 60 mm Hg. The elastic forces in the iris are transmitted to the iridocorneal angle in such a way that when the pupil is expanded, as for example with atropine, aqueous humour outflow is reduced. Carbonic anhydrase inhibitors like acetoazolamide decrease the intraocular pressure by decreasing the movement of water and electrolytes.

22. **BCD**
Surfactant is a lipoprotein produced in the type II alveolar cells. Its main role is to decrease the surface tension at the alveolar air interface. In addition pulmonary surfactant increases the mean radius of the alveoli. These two effects increase lung compliance. Normal surfactant also reduces the transpulmonary pressure that maintains lung volume and this in turn decreases the filtration forces across the pulmonary capillary.

23. **ABD**   *A must be wrong*
Iron, largely in the ferrous form, is transported into the intestinal epithelial cells where it is incorporated into ferritin, a protein iron complex which functions as an intracellular store of iron. Some of the absorbed iron is released from the cell into the plasma. Most iron is transported in the plasma bound to a polypeptide called transferrin or siderophilin. This polypeptide has two iron binding sites and is normally 35% saturated with iron.

24. **BD**
The pulmonary pressure varies from the apex to the base of the lung within the intact thorax when exposed to gravity. The apical alveoli are distended to 85–90% of their maximal volume whereas the basal alveoli contain only 35–40% of their maximal volume. The basal alveoli have a higher compliance and change their volume most over the respiratory cycle. It is the force of gravity not the pleural pressure gradient which causes the uneven blood flow distribution. The ventilation perfusion ratio increases from base to apex.

25. **E**
X-ray contrast material is freely filtered at the glomerulus, but is not secreted in the distal tubule. The contrast in renal failure is rather poor. It has been said that there is better contrast in dehydrated

subjects, but this is not the experience of many. All water soluble contrast media contain iodine.

26. AC
At menstruation there is bleeding and shedding of superficial layers. This is followed by the proliferative phase dominated by oestrogen when there is reconstruction of tissue and glands. Following ovulation is the secretory or progestational phase when the endometrium develops a rich spongy texture with oedematous swelling and vascular and glandular development.

27. AB
The renal blood flow is about 1200 ml/min some 20–25% of the cardiac output. This is very much higher than is required to provide sufficient oxygen for the kidneys even though the tubules have a high oxygen consumption. The A-V oxygen difference is thus small. The blood flow to the kidney is autoregulated so that the glomerular filtration rate remains constant over a relatively wide range of blood pressures. Some blood may be diverted away from the kidney during exercise.

28. BCD
The normal clotting time in siliconised tubes is prolonged, being 20–69 minutes, as opposed to 6–12 minutes in glass tubes. Quick's one stage test gives not only the concentration of prothrombin present in the sample, but also the concentrations of factors V, VII and X, factors participating in the activation of prothrombin. The prothrombin time is normal in haemophilia as factors VIII and IX are not required for the activation of prothrombin. Another test employed has been the thromboplastin (prothrombin activator) generation time. Intrinsic thromboplastin formation is defective in thrombocytopenia, haemophilia, Christmas disease and in hypo-prothrombinaemia. Clot retraction is normal in patients with haemophilia, but abnormal in patients with thrombocytopenia.

29. BC
The percent of oxygen in respiratory gas may be determined using a Haldane apparatus in which the volume of a given sample of gas may be determined before and after oxygen is absorbed with a solution such as chromous chloride. It may also be performed using a paramagnetic oxygen analyser or mass spectrometer. The oxygen content of plasma may be determined using the Van Slyke volumetric blood gas apparatus in which oxygen is released from haemoglobin using potassium ferricyanide to convert ferrous to

ferric iron. The volume of gas liberated may be measured. Oxygen saturation may be determined by measuring absorption by blood of monochromatic light of wavelength 630×10^{-9} m. The partial pressure of oxygen may be measured using a micro gas analysis apparatus such as the Roughton Scholander apparatus in which a bubble of gas is allowed to come into equilibrium with the blood. Oxygen electrodes - platinum electrodes may be used to measure gas tensions directly.

30. ACD

A peristaltic wave down the oesophagus aids in the movement of food towards the stomach. In the proximal stomach the major form of motility is tonic contraction while in the distal stomach vigorous peristalsis, retropulsion and chymification occur. Peristalsis may occur in the small intestine, travelling anally. The predominant movements in the large intestine are haustration and mass movements.

31. D

In the adult human at rest with mind wandering the most prominent component of the EEG is a fairly regular pattern of waves at a frequency of 8–12 per second, the alpha rhythm. The frequency is decreased by a low blood glucose concentration, a low body temperature, low levels of adrenal glucocorticoid hormones and a high partial pressure of carbon dioxide. It is increased by the reverse conditions. Forced ventilation to lower arterial PCO_2 is sometimes used clinically to bring out latent EEG abnormalities. When the eyes are opened the alpha rhythm is replaced by fast irregular lower voltage activity with no dominant frequency. This alpha block may also be produced by mental concentration such as solving arithmetic problems.

32. AC

Voluntary hyperpnoea results in reduced alveolar and arterial PCO_2. This raises the ratio of bicarbonate ions to carbon dioxide content with an accompanying increase in blood pH. Since carbon dioxide is one of the main factors influencing the diameter of the cerebral arterioles, a fall in arterial PCO_2 results in vasoconstriction and reduced oxygen availability to the brain tissue. Although CO_2 has vascular effects, arterial hypertension is not seen.

33. BE

Reduced distensibility of the arterial walls leads to an increase in the velocity of the arterial pulse wave as the vibration travels more rapidly in a stiff structure. There is also a greater rise in the magnitude of the pulse wave. The lack of elastic recoil means that the cardiac output is less readily accommodated in systole with a rise in blood pressure and that diastolic pressure tends to fall. Wall stiffness does not however affect the peripheral resistance.

34. ABC
When the sole of the foot of a normal subject is stroked, plantarflexion is seen, the so-called negative Babinski response. In the weeks and months following spinal transection motor reflexes recover. Flexor responses become more pronounced including those of the great toe. The foot, especially the sole is the most sensitive reflexogenic zone and even non-painful stimuli are sufficient to trigger flexor reflexes. Extension of the opposite leg is the crossed extensor reflex. The muscles controlling the toe will be completely paralysed in a lower motor lesion.

35. ABCD
One of the metabolic responses to surgery is retention of sodium, resulting from a number of factors. It may also be produced by administration of glucocorticoids, which have mineralocorticoid activity also. Increased vasopressin secretion however leads to hyponatraemia. Sodium retention results in relative expansion of the extracellular fluid as sodium is largely extracellular. There is also a rise in capillary blood pressure which causes oedema.

36. BC
On inspiration the lung volume increases rapidly and the alveolar pressure becomes negative producing a pressure gradient that allows respiratory flow. Pleural pressure, which at the end of expiration is about -5 cm water becomes more negative on inspiration and on expiration becomes less negative or even positive on forced pleural pressure changes as a function of both resistance and elastic forces. The major component of the resistance forces is airway resistance, the tissue resistance contributing only about 10–20% of the total. The elastance forces of the lungs can be estimated at the end of inspiration because the elastance forces are normally zero at this time.

37. A
The basal requirements of a man of surface area 1.8 m^2 is approximately 7,300 kJ. The rate of metabolism will be equal to the basal level during the 8 h of sleep. During the waking hours additional calories are required for the various activities. If this

additional requirement is assumed to be 4,400 kJ, then 11,700 kJ are required per day. This could be provided by, for example

100g fat	38 kJ/g	3,800 kJ
375g carbohydrate	17 kJ/g	6,200 kJ
100g protein	17 kJ/g	1,700 kJ
		Total 11,700 kJ

38. BC   *Anatomical + physiol should be equal !*

An anatomical shunt results in reduced arterial oxygen. This may involve a right to left shunt through septal defects in the heart, pulmonary arterial venous anastomoses or blood flow through atelectatic lungs. A physiological shunt, which is normally 1–2% of the cardiac output, represents that blood from the myocardium and bronchial tree draining back into the systemic circulation and is not oxygenated in the lungs. The administration of 100% oxygen may be used to distinguish between anatomical and physiological shunts. Administration of 100% to a patient with an anatomical shunt does not raise the PaO_2 to normal (greater than 600 mm Hg), but can increase the oxygen content of arterial blood.

B false , E correct

39. BE

There is always a small loss of fluid from the pulmonary capillaries. Fluid escaping from capillaries does not necessarily mean movement of fluid into the alveoli. This only occurs when pressure increases and increased lymph flow cannot adequately remove the fluid. Loss of fluid from the pulmonary capillary as in any other is increased by capillary pressure, but is not influenced by blood flow. Additionally in the lungs surface tension forces tend to 'suck' fluid out of the capillaries, an effect counteracted by surfactant.

40. AD

Intracranial pressure rises in a number of situations including the Valsalva manoeuvre when venous return is impaired and cerebral venous pressure is raised. Reduced CO_2 causes cerebral vasoconstriction, reduced blood volume and intracranial pressure. Increased intracranial pressure may result in the damage of a variety of cranial nerves leading to squinting and loss of the sensation of smell. It produces bulging of the disc, but in the opposite direction, papilloedema due to compression of the veins which drain from the retinal circulation and accompanying retinal nerves. Removal of the cerebrospinal fluid by lumbar puncture may cause a fatal compression of the medulla as it is coned down into the foramen magnum.

41. BD

Aldosterone is a C18 steroid hormone with a CHO residue in position 18. It is produced exclusively in the zona glomerulosa of the adrenal cortex. The main site of action of aldosterone is the distal tubule of the kidney where it increases sodium reabsorption, so promoting the retention of sodium. The sodium is exchanged for potassium and hydrogen ions in the renal tubules producing a potassium diuresis and an increase in urinary acidity.

42. AD

To compare means of independent samples the t test may be used. The distribution of t was worked out by Gosset who in 1908, under the pseudonym of Student, wrote on the distribution of t, later to be known as Student's t test. The paired t test is used for testing the significance of a change when observations are made, for example, before or after a manoeuvre in the same subject. The Mann Whitney U-test and the Wilcoxan matched pairs signed rank test are used for comparing medians.

43. ACDE

Atropine blocks the action of cholinergic constrictor fibres causing dilation of the pupil. Also blocked are the nerves supplying the ciliary muscles so that the individual has problems in focussing on near objects. The dilation of the pupil causes obstruction by the iris of the cornea and a reduction in the rate of aqueous humour outflow. Thus atropine should not be used when glaucoma, a pathological increase in the intraocular pressure, is suspected.

44. ABD

Adrenaline is synthesised in the chromaffin cells of the adrenal medulla. Synthesis starts from the essential amino acid tyrosine. It is converted to L-dopa via the action of tyrosine hydroxylase. Dopa is then decarboxylated (dopadecarboxylase) to form dopamine. These steps take place in the cytoplasm. Noradrenaline is then formed in vesicles or granules, dopamine hydroxylase being the enzyme involved. Finally the formation of adrenaline from noradrenaline occurs by the action of the enzyme phenylethano-lamine transferase, the step requiring a methyl donor such as methionine. *Phenylalanine as well!*

45. CD

Treatment with long-term corticosterone therapy in doses in excess of 7.5 mg per day results in suppression of the adrenopituitary axis. On withdrawal of therapy the symptoms observed are not improved by ACTH administration. Pituitary ACTH secretion recovers before adrenocortical responsiveness. Alternate day drug therapy has a number of advantages including the fact that certain desired pharmacological effects, for example anti-inflammatory or immunosuppressive effects, may persist for 48 h whereas undesirable actions, such as those associated with iatrogenic Cushing's syndrome, may have a shorter duration of action.

46. **ABCD**   *A: false , B: what is close ? for heavens sake*
The chemical description is 2 chloro-1,1,2 tri flouroethyl diflouromethyl ether, its boiling point is 56.6°C close to the 50.0°C of halothane. It has a muscle relaxant action partly via the central nervous system and partly by a post junctional effect, not reversed by neostigmine. 80% is excreted unchanged in the expired gas, 2–5% is metabolised in the liver. The MAC of enflurane is 1.60, that of halothane is 0.75.

47. **CDE**
Tremor has not been reported with nifedipine. They are negative inotropes. Rapid and complete absorption occurs from the sublingual route. It relaxes arteriolar smooth muscle and decreases coronary vascular resistance, producing its major effects in the treatment of angina pectoris and hypertension.

48. **ACDE**
Topical anticholinesterase to the eye causes miosis by constriction of the sphincter pupilae muscles, loss of accommodation is brought about by cilary muscle spasm. There is no effect on tear production. Conjunctival hyperaemia occurs.

49. **AB**
Dantrolene reduces the contraction of skeletal muscles by a direct action on the excitation contraction coupling. It produces muscle weakness, which limits its use as an antispasmodic drug. It is the drug of choice in treatment of malignant hyperpyrexia. It will potentiate myoneural blocking drugs. It has no effect on opiate receptors, an analeptic agent produces convulsions and muscular rigidity, e.g. strychnine, the opposite effect of dantrolene.

50. **BCDE**
The headache associated with GTN is caused by arteriolar dilatation. However generalised venodilatation lowers left and right end diastolic pressure, and pulmonary artery pressure, and transient coronary vasodilatation.

51. ~~BCE~~ *BCE*

Codeine reduces intestinal tone and causes constipation. Cimetidine has been reported as causing both diarrhoea and constipation. Phenytoin does not have any affect on the gut. Both magnesium sulphate and dioctyl sodium sulphosuccinate are used as laxatives.

52. BCE *C? if given iv. doesn't pass BBB!*

Dopamine is a positive inotrope, in doses up to 5 ml/kg/h it increases renal blood flow. It is a central nervous system transmitter, and also has an agonist action at β-receptors, and at dopaminergic receptors.

53. AE

Noradrenaline has its action terminated by neuronal uptake, and acetylcholinesterase terminates the action of acetylcholine. Diamine oxidase is better known as monoamine oxidase, choline acetyltransferase is involved in the synthesis of acetylcholine. Butrylcholinesterase is one of the plasma cholinesterase enzymes, not involved in transmitter limitation.

54. E

Streptomycin has a clearance about two thirds of GFR because of active tubular reabsorption. Penicillin on the other hand has a renal clearance equal to the total renal plasma flow, because it is actively secreted into the tubule. Chloramphenicol is largely metabolised, 25% is excreted unchanged, but its high protein binding limits its glomerular filtration. Septrin is a combination of trimethoprin and sulfamethoxazole, each with a clearance less than GFR. In the case of gentamicin there is a linear relationship between clearance and plasma level.

55. BCE

Lignocaine is an amide and withstands autoclaving. Like prilocaine the metabolism can produce methaemoglobinaemia, and toxic doses can cause central excitation and convulsions. It should never be given with adrenaline in the treatment of dysrhythmias. Both lignocaine and quinidine are class one drugs in the Vaughn-Williams classification, although they differ in their effect on the refractory period.

56. AC

Atropine blocks cholinergic receptors on bronchial smooth muscle. Ephedrine is a sympathomimetic amine. Tubocurarine can cause bronchoconstriction by histamine release, oxprenolol is a non-selective β blocker so can cause bronchoconstriction.

57. ABCDE

Morphine increases tone in the biliary tree and spasm of the sphincter. It raises arterial PCO_2 by depressing the respiratory centre. It is said to increase ADH secretion although this is controversial as to its significance. Histamine release is a common feature of morphine administration.

58. BDE

Increasing depth of enflurane anaesthesia (5–7%) can cause twitching movements, which disappear with further increase in depth of anaesthesia. Metoclopramide and droperidol in overdose can produce Parkinsonian-type movements. Neither ketamine or benzodiazepines cause involuntary movements.

59. AE

Oxytocin increases the force of uterine contractions, it causes dilatation of blood vessels and hypotension, but not arrythmias. Nausea is not a feature, indeed it has few side effects, this being its major advantage over ergotamine.

→ But it is controversial

60. D All β-Blockers increase peripheral resistance → cold feet!

Propranolol increases airways resistance, reduces the force of contraction of the myocardium, and stimulates the secretion of renin. Propran. reduces renin release

61. ABD

Suxamethonium is a dicholine ester with two quaternary ammonium groups:

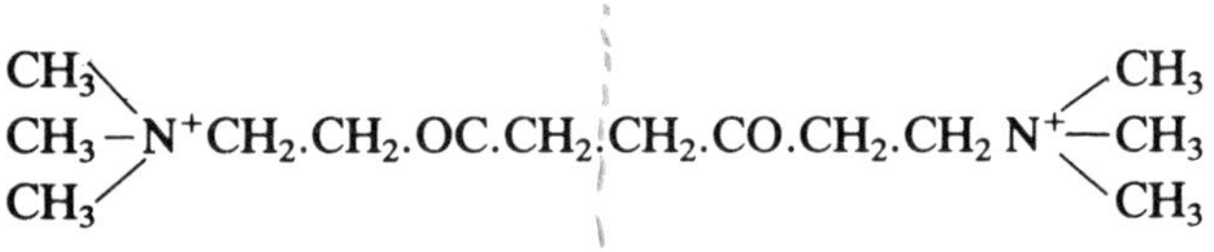

Acetylcholine is:

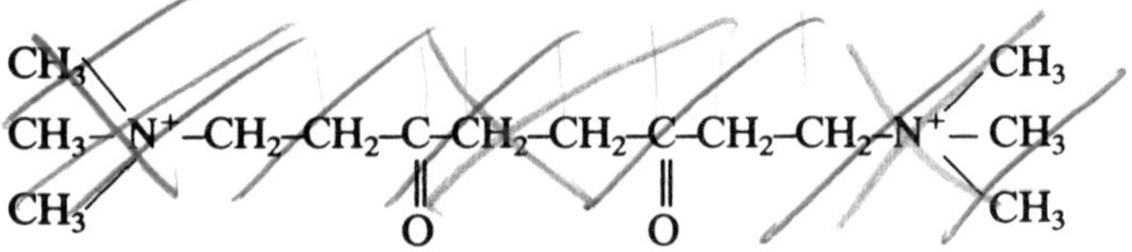

It is primarily metabolised by serum cholinesterase to succinyl choline which is then metabolised to choline and succinic acid by acetylcholinesterase. It is potentiated by a factor of two by

ACh $CH_3-CO-O-CH_2-CH_2-N^+(CH_3)_3$

neostigmine, is unstable in solution at room temperature, and is stored at 4°C.

62. ABCD
The order of producing respiratory depression is enflurane > isoflurane > halothane. The blood gas solubility of isoflurane is 1.4. All volatile agents produce cerebral vasodilation. Isoflurane does not sensitise the myocardium to catecholamines.

63. DE
Metabolism may result in more potent metabolites, it is affected by changes in liver blood flow, it frequently involves cytochrome P450. Genetic factors determine the rate of metabolism of a number of drugs.

64. AC
The butyrophenones block the action of apomorphine at dopaminergic receptors in the chemoreceptor trigger zone. They have very little peripheral action and are cardiovascularly stable; the phenothiazines, which are closely related, do act peripherally but their action is in fact anti-muscarinic in nature. When used without analgesics they can induce a state of 'inner anxiety' where hallucinations may be masked by an outer appearance of calm. They do not depress respiration, but have a higher incidence of Parkinsonian side effects than phenothiazines.

65. AB *The carbonic anhydrase inhibitor is Azetazolamide (Diamox R)*
Diazoxide is chemically related to the thiazides, and produces its antihypertensive effect by its capacity to relax arteriolar smooth muscle directly. It causes hyperglycaemia, has no α blocking action and does not release histamine.

66. ACDE
Glucagon acts as a positive inotrope via its ability to stimulate production of cyclic AMP. Vagal stimulation produces no effect on the force of contraction. Adrenaline is an α and β agonist, and isoprenaline is a β agonist. Ephedrine has both direct and indirect sympathomimetic actions.

67. AB
Phenylzine and transcypramine are monoamine oxidase inhibitors. Amitriptyline and imipramine are tricyclic antidepressants, flupenthixol is a phenothiazine related compound with anti-depressive properties.

68. AB

Clonidine is a central α_2 agonist which produces a reduction in systolic, mean and diastolic blood pressure, and in heart rate. Rebound hypertension occurs and may be difficult to treat. Its action is confined to the α_2 receptor, and it has no action on angiotensin.

69. AC

Established triggers for malignant hyperpyrexia are suxamethonium and all volatile anaesthetic agents. Psychotropic drugs are also under suspicion, but it may be that the neourolept malignant syndrome is a different entity. Opioids, local anaesthetics, competitive muscle relaxants, and nitrous oxide are apparently safe.

70. AC

Imipramine and amitryptiline are tricyclic antidepressants, and have their action by preventing re-uptake of noradrenaline into nerve endings. Dopamine is a sympathetic and dopaminergic agonist, carbamizole is an anti thyroid drug, and isocarboxazid is a monoamine oxidase inhibitor.

71. DE

Increasing lipid solubility decreases duration of action, as redistribution is more rapid. Epileptics are not particularly sensitive to barbiturates. The concurrent ingestion of other CNS depressants is additive. The barbiturates are all to a greater or lesser extent protein bound, so hypoalbuminaemia will increase the proportion of free drug and potentiate it. Alkalisation of the urine keeps weak acids ionised in the urine.

72. BCE

Plasma cholinesterase is synthesised in the liver, it hydrolyses specifically choline esters, and it is confined to the plasma. Sodium fluoride is used as an inhibitor in one of the tests of abnormal cholinesterases. It can be congenitally absent, although suxamethonium apnoea is in most cases due to abnormal enzyme.

73. ACDE

Salbutamol is a β agonist, and as such it causes bronchodilation tachycardia and relaxes the pregnant uterus. It is well absorbed via the aerosol route, as can be seen by the tachycardia which often accompanies the use of aerosol salbutamol. Like isoprenaline it does not affect the pulmonary artery pressure.

74. BDE

Ketamine, etomidate, and suxamethonium are all dissolved in water, although etomidate also has 35% propylene glycol present. Propanidid is dissolved in polyoxyethylated castor oil and althesin was dissolved in cremophor EL.

75. ACD ~~*D → increases LOS. Pharma book P 526*~~

Metoclopramide is antidopaminergic, and prolactin secretion is suppressed by dopamine. It has no effect on blood pressure, and is anti-emetic. Although rare, dystonia and other Parkinsonian side effects can occur. Lowering of the lower oesophageal tone is brought about by the systemic cholinergic action.

76. ACD

Atropine blocks the vagus allowing sympathetic tone to increase the heart rate. Pancuronium causes sympathetic stimulation resulting in tachycardia. Gallamine has an atropine-like effect on the vagus. Vecuronium does not block the vagus in clinically useful doses, it has no effect on the heart rate. Fentanyl is a potent opioid and its use is often associated with a bradycardia.

77. ABCDE

Lignocaine causes convulsions in toxic doses, insulin via hypoglycaemia, and oxygen as part of its acute toxicity. Nikethamide and amphetamine are both CNS stimulants.

78. DE

Naloxone is an antagonist at all opioid receptors. The vomiting induced by morphine is due to a direct effect on the chemoreceptor trigger zone and not via an opioid receptor therefore it is not reversed by naloxone. It has been shown to increase blood pressure in animals with induced hypovolaemic shock, and a few reports indicate it may be of benefit in patients. Pentazocine is an agonist-antagonist and can have its actions partially reversed by naloxone.

79. ABCE *1.15*

Unlike halothane and enflurane, isoflurane does not sensitise the myocardium to catecholamines. Its minimum alveolar concentration (MAC) is ~~0.75~~ in the absence of nitrous oxide, 0.29 in 70% nitrous oxide. It is the least metabolised of the halogenated volatile agents. It reduces the systemic vascular resistance despite which liver blood flow is maintained.

not any more:
Desflurane = 0.02%

137

80. D
Labetolol is a drug with both α and β blocking actions, the β blocking action is more long lasting than the α blocking.

PRACTICE EXAM 4

1. ABCE
Vagal stimulation directly increases gastrin output. The hormone is also released on entry of food into the stomach. Two mechanisms may be involved, the distension which triggers the vagal reflex and the products of digestion which act as secretagogues. Gastrin release is also regulated by feedback inhibition, the crucial stimulus being pH. Thus the buffer action of food when it enters the stomach produces a rise in pH and gastrin secretion. As well as stimulating gastric secretion, gastrin produces an increase in gastric blood flow.

2. AC
The bicarbonate buffer system is probably the most effective in the body. The pH of the interstitial fluid is well above the pK of the bicarbonate buffer system, but it is a volatile buffer system in which the bicarbonate is in equilibrium with CO_2. Protein also represents an effective buffer in the body. There is little protein in the interstitial or cerebrospinal fluid and the bicarbonate buffer pair is the main buffer system. The main buffer of the red cells is haemoglobin and that of the cells probably protein. When increasing numbers of hydrogen ions pass into the urine they are largely excreted as ammonium ions.

3. ABD
Cardiac output depends on the heart rate and the stroke volume. A rise in the body temperature increases the heart rate acting directly on the pacemaker (S-A node) and also on the cardiac centre. Stroke volume depends on the contractility of the heart, which in turn depends on a number of factors influencing the activity of the sympathetic nervous system and the venous return. Gravity hinders the return of blood from the dependent parts and therefore raising the legs improves venous return. Contraction of muscles forces flow of blood back to the heart, the process being aided by the presence of the valves in the veins. On inspiration the pressure in the thorax falls to about -8 mm Hg and even more (-30 mm Hg) on exercise which aids return of the blood to the heart. This respiratory pump action is lost in open chest surgery.

4. **ABCE**
Hypoxia in anaemia is due to haemoglobin deficiency; in stagnant hypoxia it is due to slow circulation in organs such as the kidney and heart and histotoxic hypoxia to inhibition of tissue oxidative processes. In these conditions the arterial concentration can be raised only slightly by increasing the amount of oxygen in physical solution. This is also true of hypoxic hypoxia resulting from shunting of oxygenated blood past the lungs. In other forms of hypoxia oxygen administration may be of great benefit. However in some patients the carbon dioxide level may be so high that it is only the hypoxic drive which maintains respiration.

5. **ABCE**
The formation of tissue fluid is dependent on the balance between the hydrostatic forces and the oncotic pressure of the plasma. Any condition which increases net filtration will produce oedema. Such conditions are those in which there is a fall in plasma protein concentration such as renal failure or Kwashiorkor, the syndrome which can develop when a child is weaned. Increased interstitial fluid formation is also seen with increased hydrostatic pressure on the arterial or venous side as seen in heart failure. It is not seen in myxoedema in which there is reduced secretion of thyroid hormones.

6. **A**
Basal metabolic rate, the energy required under basal conditions, may be measured indirectly by calorimetry. The oxygen uptake of an individual is determined using a spirometer and from this the calories produced may be calculated. The average value for men is 170 kJ (40 kcal) per m^2 per hour and that for women 155 kJ (37 kcal). It is higher in children and reduced in tropical climates. It is influenced by thyroid hormones, being increased in hyperthyroidism and decreased in hypothyroidism. Thus it is usually elevated in patients with Graves' disease. However goitre is also found in hypothyroid patients.

7. **ABC**
Airway resistance is given by $P/V = P_{alv}/R$. To determine airway resistance, one must measure the pressure difference between the mouth and alveoli and the simultaneous flow rate. An indirect procedure employing the body plethysmography is used. When the system is calibrated the change in pressure in the chamber can be measured at the same time using a pneumotachograph. Alternatively measurement may be made of the pressure/flow relationship

at the mouth when the subject is connected to a source of forced air oscillations from a loudspeaker. Another method used is to subtract from the total pressure generating flow, the component required to overcome elastic resistance, thus leaving the component required to overcome non-elastic resistance.

8. **BDE**

   Iron absorption from the intestine is an active process occurring most rapidly in the upper small intestine. It is facilitated by conversion of dietary iron from the ferric form (Fe^{3+}) to the ferrous (Fe^{2+}) form. This is aided by the low gastric pH which favours reduction and is also facilitated by the presence of reducing substances such as vitamin C. Some of the absorbed iron passes to the blood stream, but most is bound to a protein apoferritin in the cell to form ferritin. This is a major storage form of iron in the body. This iron is in equilibrium with that bound to transferrin in the plasma. Iron is also released from the mucosal cells according to the body's need for iron as expressed in the plasma iron or the extent of transfusion saturation.

9. **ABCD**

   If the demand for increased effort by the heart is repeated, as in athletes or continuous, as when the heart has to pump against a high systemic blood pressure, the heart enlarges. In athletes the enlargement of the heart up to 500 g, as compared with a normal mass of 300 g, is seen in those specialising in long term performance. As the hypertrophy develops in a chronically loaded heart, the number of myocardial cells at first is constant while the length and thickness increases. Once the hypertrophied heart reaches a critical mass (above 500 g) hyperplasia develops in which the size and number of the fibres increases. The oxygen consumption is greater in chronically dilated hearts with a danger of angina. The ECG can be used only to determine electrical changes in the heart.

10. **C**

    The main site of resistance in the vascular system is the arteriolar bed, the drop across the capillaries being relatively smaller. Thus the greatest drop of about 70–75 mm Hg is seen on passing from the femoral artery to the vein. The drop from the aorta to the brachial artery is only a few mm Hg, that across the capillary bed about 20 mm Hg and that from the saphenous artery to the right atrium also about 20 mm Hg. The pressure in the pulmonary artery is only about 15 mm Hg, so again the pressure drop is not as great as in the systemic circulation.

11. CD +E (Harvey)

Obligatory absorption of salt and water equivalent to about 7/8 of the filtered load occurs in the proximal tubule. The fluid reabsorbed is isotonic with plasma as is the fluid remaining in the tubule. While sodium is actively reabsorbed across the luminal membrane of the proximal tubule, chloride is passively absorbed along an electrochemical gradient. PAH, which is virtually completely cleared in one passage through the kidney is actively secreted at this site, but not potassium. In reabsorption of bicarbonate, hydrogen ions are secreted into the tubular fluid where they combine with the filtered bicarbonate to form carbonic acid from which CO_2 is formed and water. The CO_2 diffuses into the tubular cell, where under the influence of carbonic anhydrase, carbonic acid and hence bicarbonate for reabsorption is formed.

12. ABCE

Pituitary tumours can be treated in a number of ways, including hypophysectomy. Such a technique has been used in the treatment of acromegaly and gigantism. Total hypophysectomy often causes remission of the disease but is a very specialised technique necessitating permanent replacement for hypopituitarism. Partial hypophysectomy may be performed for extrasellar extensions involving visual pathways. Selective removal of the adenoma may sometimes be achieved leaving behind normally functioning tissue. The patient may be left with gonadotrophin or other pituitary deficiencies, diabetes insipidus, c.s.f. rhinorrhoea or meningitis.

13. ABDE

Dark adaptation is an increase in the eye's sensitivity when kept in darkness. Dark adaptation has two phases, an initial rapid phase reflecting the increase in cone sensitivity and a slower phase reflecting the increase in rod sensitivity. However photochemical adaptation does not occur to the same extent in cones as in rods, which is why rods function primarily at night. The process involves an increase in the concentration of photosensitive pigments.

14. BCD

The normal blood volume at birth is about 90 ml/kg and the cardiac output per minute can exceed this. The oxygen consumption is about twice that of the adult on a weight basis and the respiratory rate is double. As compared with the adult the kidney has a relatively low ability to regulate osmolality, volume and acid base balance. Vasopressin is secreted at birth, but there is a relatively low capacity to concentrate the urine because there is an inadequate development of the countercurrent mechanism and decreased sensitivity of the tubular cells to vasopressin.

15. C

Coronary blood flow occurs mainly during diastole and is stopped during the height of systole due to compression of the vessels by contraction of the ventricular muscle. There is vasodilatation on injection of adrenaline and also during hypotension which causes an increase in the adrenergic stimulus. In congestive heart failure there is an increase in venous pressure leading to a reduction in effective coronary perfusion and hence a decrease in coronary blood flow.

16. ABDE

Oxygen consumption may be determined using a spirometer with a carbon dioxide absorber and bell. The rate of decrease of volume directly indicates the volume of oxygen consumed. Depending on the body size, oxygen consumption per minute is 520 ml, equivalent to about 5 kJ (240 kcal/min). On exercise ventilation increases linearly. Hyperventilation at rest increases the oxygen consumption only slightly, so a smaller fraction of oxygen is removed from the much larger volume of inspired gas. Therefore oxygen in the expired air increases.

~250 mls/min

17. AE

Deuterium (D_2O) and tritium oxide readily cross cell membranes and are evenly distributed throughout the body as is urea. The degree of dilution of D_2O or tritium oxide following intravenous injection allows calculation of total body water. Evans blue binds to plasma albumin and so is retained in the cardiovascular system and may be used to determine plasma volume. Potassium is largely intracellular, its concentration being maintained by the sodium/potassium pump and the differential permeability of the membrane. Insulin does not enter the cells, acting at receptors in the plasma membrane.

18. C

Myogenic tone describes the contractions seen in smooth muscle which results from spontaneous electrical activity. The appropriate term for the activity in the nerves supplying vascular smooth muscle is vasomotor tone and that for the maintained contraction seen in the absence of electrical activity is contracture. The activity seen in postural muscles is dependent on neural activity.

19. **BC**
    Erythropoietin as its name implies stimulates erythropoiesis, doing so by enhancing the proliferation of erythrocyte precursor cells in bone marrow. The exact structure of the hormone is unknown but it is a sialo-protein with a molecular weight of 46,000. The primary source is the kidney although it may be produced in the liver. Erythropoietin is elevated by conditions that create tissue hypoxia. It is also increased in states with increased need for oxygen such as hyperthyroidism.

20. **ABDE**
    The amount of oxygen carried in the blood to a given organ per unit of time is the product of the arterial oxygen concentration (O_2) and the rate of blood flow (Q)

    O_2 availability $= O_2$ x Q

    The oxygen concentration can be derived from the saturation (SO_2) on the basis of Hufner's number as follows:

    $O_2 = 1.34$ x Hb x SO_2 x 10 - 5

    The relationship first described implies that differences in the availability of oxygen to the various organs are entirely ascribable to differences in blood flow through the organs. Any change in blood flow as a result of changes in vascular resistance or mean arterial pressure results directly in a change in the amount of oxygen available to the tissue.

21. **B**
    Artificial ventilation may be administered using positive pressure respirators which inflate the lungs by cyclically blowing air into them. Expiration may be brought about by the pressure recoil of the lung and chest wall. Alternatively a negative pressure phase may be incorporated in the pump so that expired air is sucked out. The increase in the intrathoracic pressure on inspiration impairs the venous return and in turn the cardiac output.

22. **ACDE**
    The terminal ileum is the main site of absorption of bile salts which are essential for absorption of fats. They are secreted by the liver in the bile, pass into the gastro-intestinal tract, where they aid in the absorption not only of fats but also of fat soluble vitamins A,D,E, and K. Deficiency of vitamin A leads to night blindness and of

vitamin K to bleeding tendencies. Vitamin B_{12} is absorbed only from the terminal ileum, so that resection of the ileum results in megaloblastic anaemia. Iron absorption occurs largely in the upper small intestine, so iron deficiency anaemia is not seen.

23. **CE**

    Parathyroid hormone secretion is stimulated by a low plasma calcium, as occurs in chronic renal failure, and also by an acute fall in plasma magnesium. A fall in plasma phosphate would be associated with an increase in plasma calcium as would administration of vitamin D and hence a fall in plasma parathyroid hormone. The demineralisation of bone seen in patients after prolonged immobilisation results not from alterations in parathyroid hormone secretion, but in a reduction in the mechanical stresses applied to bone.

24. **E**

    After a clot is formed serum is expressed and the clot becomes smaller – clot retraction. This process depends on intact platelets. In some manner the platelets exert tension on the fibrin strands. Disintegrated platelets have no effect; neither are leucocytes, nor erythrocytes involved in the process. Factor VIII is involved in blood coagulation rather than clot retraction. Deficiency of factor VIII results in haemophilia.

25. **ACDE**

    The adrenal gland is a composite of mesodermal ridge in the dorsal abdominal cavity (cortex) and a modified sympathetic ganglion i.e. neural crest (medulla); hence the secretion of adrenaline. Both the pigment cells in the skin and retina develop directly from the brain –the optic vesicles, while all other pigment cells come from the wandering neural crest. The Schwann cells are also derived from the neural crest.

26. **CDE**

    A pneumothorax may result from a ruptured alveolus, an incision through the chest wall or an injection of air through the chest wall. When it occurs, because of the characteristic elastic recoil of the lungs, the residual volume is reduced. The presence of air in the intrapleural space would tend to reduce the normal inward pull of the lung on the chest wall, making the wall tend to expand. The intrapleural pressure moves away from subatmospheric towards atmospheric and there is a damping of pressure changes. There is a lower intrathoracic pressure on the normal side which tends to pull the mediastinum to that side.

27. **CDE**

A low plasma potassium does not reflect a fall in body potassium. It may be due to vomiting as a result of the loss of cells from the epithelium or to enhanced potassium secretion resulting from alkalosis. Aldosterone deficiency would result in potassium retention. Low plasma potassium interferes with the activity of smooth muscle and may cause paralytic ileus. At low extracellular potassium contractions the stimulating activity on pacemaker activity dominates and cardiac arrhythmias are seen.

28. **ABE**

In the first stage of acute renal failure urinary output dips below 700 ml/24 h. Complete anuria is unusual except in the case of obstruction of the urinary tract. There is a failure to concentrate urine and urea and potassium released from cell breakdown accumulate in the plasma. Urinary urea is below 175 mmol/l. The failure to excrete hydrogen ions causes an acidosis with a fall in plasma bicarbonate. The chief danger is cardiac arrest due to hyperkalaemia.

29. **BCE**

Inputs from the chemoreceptors contribute to the control of respiration, the central chemoreceptors responding to CO_2 being the more important. As with other reflex pathways in the central nervous system that involved in stimulation of respiration on hypercapnia is depressed. The response to hypoxia is better maintained and this may account for most of the respiratory drive. Oxygen administration may then remove the drive and lead to CO_2 retention. The latter is observed as anaesthesia deepens leading to a fall in pH. Spontaneous ventilation ceases when the respiratory centre is sufficiently depressed by anaesthesia.

30. **ADE**

Haemoglobin is synthesised in erythrocyte precursors. In the early embryo, blood formation takes place first in the mesoderm of the yolk sac. After the third month of fetal life synthesis takes place primarily in the fetal liver and spleen. After the middle of fetal life the bone marrow begins to act as a blood forming organ. By 20 years of age the femur and tibia have stopped producing erythrocytes and thereafter they are produced in the sternum, ribs and sacrum.

31. **CE**

Androgens are normally found in the circulation of the normal adult female, producing growth of axillary and pubic hair. They are secreted together with other steroids from the adrenal cortex. They may be secreted in relatively large quantities from tumours producing a number of changes involving enlargement of the clitoris and a deepening of the voice due to enlargement of the larynx. There is a failure to menstruate as androgens antagonise the effects of oestrogen on the endometrium.

32. ABC
The parasympathetic nerves are concerned with promoting vegetative functions, so that stimulation of these nerves would produce elevated secretions and increased motility of the gastro-intestinal tract. Loss of vagal inputs would result in decreased production of saliva and enzymes and decreased motility of the stomach and intestine. Nervous stimulation does not directly affect absorption and so protein absorption is not altered.

33. CDE
Cirrhosis is associated with a reduced synthesis of plasma proteins including thyroxine binding globulin. The reduced plasma protein production together with the portal hypertension leads to ascites. Accumulation of fluid in the peritoneal cavity reduces the effective body fluid volume and compensatory mechanisms to retain body fluid come into operation and lead in turn to ascites. These include increased secretion of aldosterone and vasopressin.

34. BC
On destruction of myelin the nodes of Ranvier disappear and conduction will not be saltatory. There is no lateral conduction of activity. Even if the myelin is lost, the axon still has a cell membrane, so potassium is not lost.

35. CDE
Upward displacement of the diaphragm during pregnancy might be expected to reduce the vital capacity, but in fact the diminished height of the pleural cavity is compensated for by an increase in width so that the vital capacity is unchanged. Tidal volume and pulmonary ventilation are increased in pregnancy. This may be due to a greater sensitivity of the respiratory centre to CO_2 and results in a fall in PCO_2 by about 1 kPa (7 mm Hg). This may be an effect of progesterone. The alkalosis may contribute to the placental transfer of gases. The double Bohr effect aids the uptake of O_2 by the fetal blood.

36. ABC

Blood shows anomolous viscosity, that is it does not behave as a Newtonian fluid, the viscosity of which is independent of shear. Viscosity depends on the components of the blood, namely the packed cell volume, the plasma, and the protein content in particular, although it is little affected by very small variations in protein. It is influenced by temperature, being increased by a fall in temperature. Viscosity is increased in burns, being associated with fluid loss and increased erythrocyte aggregation. Viscosity decreases in vessels of very small diameter, probably due to plasma streaming. Viscosity also depends on flow velocity decreasing with increases in flow rate.

37. CD

Calcium is present in lower concentrations in cytoplasm than in the extracellular fluid, being actively extruded from nerves and taken up by the sarcoplasmic reticulum of the muscle. Calcium serves to stabilise the membrane so a fall in extracellular calcium increases excitability as occurs in tetany. Calcium potentiates neurotransmitter release and in muscles provides a link between excitation and contraction. Changes in extracellular calcium do not influence the strength of contraction.

38. ABE

Following partial removal of the stomach, food intake may be reduced as the food reservoir effectively provided by the stomach is reduced. There is also malabsorption of fat due to rapid intestinal transit resulting from alterations in gastric emptying. The anaemia seen results from two causes. Gastric HCl aids in iron absorption by converting the ferric iron to the ferrous form. Intrinsic factor produced in the gastric mucosa is also needed for B_{12} absorption. The gastro-colic reflex is not essential for defaecation.

39. BCE

The basal membrane of the follicular cells contains a system for the active transport of iodide from the bloodstream into the cells against a steep iodide concentration gradient and also an electric gradient. A variety of ions with approximately the same van der Waal's radii as iodide, including thiocyanate, inhibit the pump. Synthesis of thyroid hormones is stimulated by TSH, whose activity is reproduced by thyroid stimulating antibody. Normally the output of T4 is greater than T3. The peroxidase enzyme and hence the iodination reaction is sensitive to inhibition by a number of antithyroid drugs including the thiocarbamines (e.g. thiouracil).

40. ACE
Respiratory minute work is increased with increases in the resistance of the system as seen with airway constriction. It is also increased when increased volumes of air are moved as with increased tidal volume and when the density of the air increases. Turbulence impedes flow so work is decreased with a decrease in turbulence. Similarly with an increase in compliance or reduced resistance to distension there is a decrease in respiratory minute work.

41. BCDE
Vasopressin is synthesised in the hypothalamus and packed into neurosecretory granules which are transported to the posterior pituitary from which the hormone is released. Thus the cells producing the hormone are non-myelinated neurones and release occurs in response to an action potential arising in the hypothalamus. The main physiological stimuli for vasopressin release are an increase in plasma osmolality and a fall in plasma volume, the two stimuli interacting so that the response to hypertonicity is enhanced during hypovolaemia. There are other stimuli of vasopressin release including pain. The hormone promotes antidiuresis by acting on the collecting ducts to increase the permeability to water. Being a peptide hormone, it binds with receptors in the plasma membrane and acts via a second messenger (cyclic AMP).

42. AB
The parasympathetic system has a cranial and sacral outflow from the central nervous system. The parasympathetic innervation of the internal anal sphincter is inhibitory though it is excitatory to the colonic musculature. Distension of the rectum provokes pelvic afferent impulses arising from muscle receptors in the rectal wall. These induce reflex parasympathetic discharges which inhibit the internal sphincter and inhibition of the discharge in the somatic pudendal fibres which results in relaxation of the external sphincter. The smooth muscle of the urinary bladder has a rich parasympathetic nerve supply. Stimulation of the bladder stretch receptors activates the parasympathetic nerve supply causing bladder contraction and simultaneously inhibits the somatic motor nerves innervating the external urethral sphincter resulting in urination.

43. B
The effect of aldosterone antagonists is to block the so-called exchange of sodium and potassium in the distal tubule. Thus sodium

absorption is reduced leading to increased sodium loss and a resulting increase in urine volume with a fall in blood volume and increase in osmolality and packed cell volume. Potassium retention occurs with, in some cases mild hyperkalaemia.

44. ABCE

Cortisol affects protein, carbohydrate and fat metabolism. Patients with Cushing's syndrome are protein depleted as a result of excess protein catabolism. The skin and subcutaneous tissues are thin and the muscles poorly developed. Body fat shows a characteristic distribution, the extremities are thin, but fat collects in the abdomen, face and upper back where it produces a buffalo hump. The salt and water retention together with the facial obesity give the rounded, moon faced appearance and there may be significant potassium depletion and weakness.

45. ABDE

The SD is a description of the scatter of observations which have a normal distribution. On average 66.8% of observations lie within one standard deviation of the mean and 95% within two standard deviations. Two variations of the formula are

1.96

$$\frac{\sqrt{\varepsilon(x - \bar{x})^2}}{n} \quad \text{and} \quad \frac{\sqrt{\varepsilon x^2 - \varepsilon x^2}}{n}$$

The value n-1 may be used instead of n to give a better estimate of the population from which the sample population (n observations) is drawn.

46. ABE

Isoprenaline is well absorbed from the oral mucosa and thus avoids first pass metabolism, when absorbed from the stomach most is inactivated in the liver. For this reason it is given by inhaler in asthma. It is a β agonist and not blocked by phenothiazines, it is less arrhythmogenic than adrenaline.

47. ABD

Levodopa crosses into the brain and is metabolised there to dopamine. Hyoscine is markedly sedative, but hyoscine-N-butyl bromine is ionised at pH 7.4 and does not enter the brain. Paracetamol has its action in the brain, and although 5 hydroxy-

tryptamine is a central transmitter, if given peripherally it is rapidly
hydrolysed.

48. ABE
Propofol was formally dissolved in cremophor, but was withdrawn
and reformulated in soya bean oil fat emulsion. It lowers the
systemic vascular resistance and systolic blood pressure. It has its
action terminated by redistribution but its principal metabolic
pathway is in the liver by glucuronide formation. A sleep dose in an
unpremedicated patient is approximately 2.5 mg/kg. It is more
respiratory depressant than thiopentone.

49. BD
Chlorthiazide, frusemide, and acetazolamide all cause loss of
potassium. Spironolactone is an aldosterone antagonist and spares
potassium, mannitol is an osmotic diuretic and does not affect
potassium homeostasis.

50. AB + ∋
The half life of chlorpropamide is 33 hours. Sulphonamides displace
it from protein binding sites and inhibit its metabolism, phenylbutazone also displaces it from protein binding sites. Propranolol
potentiates its activity, thiazides cause hyperglycaemia and reduce
the effect of chlorpropamide.

51. AD
Dichloralphenazone is metabolised to chloral, and prednisone to
prednisolone, both the active forms. Paracetamol is itself a
metabolite of phenacetin which was withdrawn due to toxicity, and
caffeine is the active metabolite of methylxanthine. The metabolites of phenytoin are all inactive.

52. ABC
Diazoxide decreases the secretion of insulin for up to 8 hours.
Glucagon and adrenaline antagonise insulin in their physiological
roles. Propranolol potentiates insulin and tolbutamide stimulates
the islets to secrete insulin. b decrease insulin secretion

53. A
Methohexitone is rapidly inactivated by metabolism whereas
thiopentone is inactivated by redistribution. The compound is not
isomeric, and it is an oxybarbiturate. All barbiturates are contraindicated in porphyria, and excitatory phenomena without EEG
changes do occur.

54. AD
Neostigmine is an alternative substrate for acetylcholinesterase and carbamylates the enzyme preventing it from hydrolysing acetylcholine. It does have some postjunctional effects by binding itself with receptors. Bronchial smooth muscle constricts due to increased acetylcholine, and motor activity of the large and small bowel is augmented. It intensifies depolarising block.

55. CDE
Ether causes changes in liver function but not jaundice, trichloroethylene causes cardiac failure, but not jaundice. Halothane hepatitis is now a recognised entity, chloroform is considered a true hepatotoxin, and fatal massive liver necrosis has been reported following methoxyflurane.

56. ABDE
Increasing the inspired concentration and the alveolar ventilation delivers more agent to the alveolar-blood interface. Potency of the agent will not affect the rate of uptake, but a lower minimum alveolar concentration will produce sleep. As the mixed venous tension rises the rate of entry into the blood slows and the alveolar tension rapidly approaches the inspired tension. The addition of nitrous oxide to the mixture produces the second gas effect.

57. BCDE
Fasciculations occur with depolarizing block. Neostigmine is an acetylcholinesterase inhibitor preventing the breakdown of acetylcholine. Partial block is characterised by fade and post tetanic facilitation. Metabolic acidosis always prolongs non-depolarising block. Aminoglycoside antibiotics prevent release of acetylcholine from pre junctional sites. *not true! Abaccurium breaks down faster!*

58. ABCDE
All these factors can affect the transfer of drugs across any lipid membrane.

59. BCD
Aminoglycosides do not affect bone marrow proliferation. They do not produce ataxia, although peripheral neuropathies, and the vestibular damage may combine to produce abnormalities of gait. Tinnitus, neuromuscular block via calcium channel blockade, and polyuric renal failure, via renal tubular damage, are all documented.

60. BCDE
Pentazocine is about half as potent as morphine, it blocks mu receptors in high doses, and the respiratory depression is reversible by naloxone. Hallucinations occur in doses exceeding 60 mg i.v. In low doses it is a weak antagonist at the mu receptor but a strong agonist for kappa receptors.

61. BCD
Hyoscine is more sedative than atropine. Atropine has a greater cardiac effect than hyoscine, and a greater antisialogogue effect than glycopyrrolate. It causes hyperpyrexia due to a central effect. Therapeutic doses of atropine do not completely block all actions of acetylcholine.

62. ABE
Trimetaphan and hexamethonium are ganglion blocking agents. Ouabain is a cardiac glycoside, and diphenylhydramine is an H_1 receptor blocker. Benzhexol acts largely in the CNS but has some peripheral anti-muscarinic action.

63. BCDE
Dopamine is an agonist, it reduces arteriolar resistance in the mesenteric vessels, and increases renal blood flow via dopaminergic receptors in the kidney. It is also a β agonist, increasing the cardiac output and thus decreasing the peripheral to central temperature gradient. *as a neurotransmitter, it has inhibitory function.*

64. CD
Cimetidine is an H_2 antagonist, it is highly polar and does not easily cross the placenta. It reduces both the acidity and volume of gastric secretions. It binds to cytochrome P450 and diminishes the activity of hepatic microsomal mixed function oxidases, as a result a number of drugs can accumulate if given concurrently with cimetidine. It has no action on the uterus.
But: There is a relaxing H_2 + a contraction H_1 receptor of uterus!

65. A
The role of digoxin in the treatment of arrhythmias is basically to reduce the rate by slowing A-V conduction. It is therefore appropriate in the treatment of atrial flutter, but not in any ventricular arrythmias. Cardiac tamponade should be managed surgically if it is compromising the circulation.

66. ACE
Hyoscine, perphenazine and cycline are all anti-emetics. Carbi-

mazole is an anti-thyroid drug. Apomorphine stimulates the chemoreceptor trigger zone and produces vomiting.

67. **AB**
Urine of pH <7.7 increases the excretion of salicylates. Excretion of all barbiturates, especially phenobarbitone are increased by alkaline diuresis. But that of pethidine, tricyclics and theophylline are unaffected by urinary pH.

68. **BD**
Salbutamol, a β_2 agonist reduces uterine contractions, as does alcohol. Prostaglandin $F_2\alpha$ induces strong uterine contractions as does oxytocin. Aspirin does not affect uterine contractions.

69. **BD**
Methohexitone is an oxybarbiturate, contraindicated in acute intermittent porphyria, as all barbiturates are. It is 70% protein bound, and more potent than thiopentone. It is largely metabolised in the liver.

70. **BDE**
Enflurane is a substituted methyl ethyl ether as are its isomers isoflurane and methoxyflurane. The blood gas coefficient of isoflurane is 1.4 of halothane it is 2.3. The overall systemic vascular resistance is not lowered by halothane. -, *nonsens*

71. **BC**
Chlorpromazine can cause hypersensitivity reactions in the liver, but does not induce enzymes. DDT in relatively low doses induces hepatic enzymes, as do all barbiturates. Benzodiazepines do not induce enzymes.

72. **AE**
Cephalosporins and flucloxacillin are well absorbed by mouth. Kanamycin is used in the treatment of hepatic coma by mouth for its local effects in the gut, it is however better absorbed than neomycin. Vancomycin is poorly absorbed, and carbenicillin is not available in an oral form as it is so poorly absorbed.

73. **BD**
Lipid solubility increases ease of transfer of drugs, highly ionised drugs do not pass across lipid membranes. Low molecular weight drugs transfer more easily. Dose and rate of metabolism do not affect transfer.

74. BCDE
Enflurane is non explosive in air or an air/oxygen mixture, its blood/gas coefficient is 1.9 (ether 12). High concentrations in the presence of hypocarbia cause EEG changes and seizure activity. At 1 MAC the $PaCO_2$ is higher than for any of the other volatile agents. It is an isomer of isoflurane.

75. CE
Nitrous oxide is rapidly taken up but has a low potency, MAC 105%, sleep is induced in almost hypoxic mixtures (80% +). Stage 111 anaesthesia, surgical anaesthesia, cannot be truly achieved with nitrous oxide and oxygen alone, but MAC values are additive, so it will lower the MAC of other concurrently administered agents. The cylinders contain only nitrous oxide, all contaminants are carefully removed. Bone marrow suppression can occur after long term (24 hours +) use.

76. E
Propofol is a phenolic structure, the solution formulated for clinical use is non aqueous so does not have a pH. It is formulated in soya bean oil emulsion. 40% of the drug appears in the urine as glucuronide. It can cause pain on injection.

77. ACE
Morphine commonly causes histamine induced skin rashes, and can cause bronchospasm. Gut motility is decreased, and it has no influence on blood sugar. Pentazocine is an agonist/antagonist at mu receptors and can antagonise morphine.

78. BCDE
Propranolol is a β blocker and as a result it slows the speed of A-V conduction, and the upstroke of the action potential. It has both local anaesthetic action of equivalent potency to lignocaine, and because of its non selectivity it can cause bronchoconstriction.

79. BCDE
The passage of drugs across the placenta is governed by the same principles which apply to all other membranes. Neostigmine is a quaternary amine, and is completely ionised at physiological pH so will not cross. Curare, suxamethonium, and hyoscine all cross the placenta, but in clinically insignificant amounts. Thiopentone is highly lipid soluble and crosses the placenta easily.

80. **A**

Priming with a dose of gallamine 5–20 mg may prevent the pains associated with suxamethonium. The salt used has no influence. The pains more commonly occur in women and in middle-aged patients rather than at the extremes of age. Post operative mobilisation does not influence the pains, indeed the onset of the pains can be delayed up to the fourth post operative day. The extent of visible fasciculations is not related to the subsequent severity of the symptoms.

READING AND REFERENCE BOOKS

Almost all the answers, if only searched for carefully can be found in:
Atkinson R. S., Rushman G. B. and Lee J. A. **A Synopsis of Anaesthesia** 10th edition 1987. John Wright and Sons, Bristol.

It is however true to say that no one book has all the answers and it is necessary to read and refer to a number of books to find the type of detailed information required for the Part 2 FCAnaes.

Goodman L. S. and Gilman A. **The Pharmacological Basis of Therapeutics** 1985 edition. Collier Macmillan Publishing Company.
Nimmo W. S. and Smith G. **Anaesthesia** 1989 edition. Blackwell Scientific Publications.

PHARMACOLOGY

Calvey N. and Williams N. E. **Principles and Practice of Pharmacology for Anaesthetists** 1982 edition. Blackwell Scientific Publications.
Clark B. and Smith D. A. **An Introduction to Pharmacokinetics** 2nd revised edition 1986. Blackwell Scientific Publications.

PHYSIOLOGY

Ganong W. F. **Review of Medical Physiology** 14th edition 1989. Prentis Hall International Edition.
Mountcastle V. B. **Medical Physiology** 14th edition 1980. Mosby Ltd.
West J. B. **Respiratory Physiology** 3rd edition 1985. Williams and Wilkins Ltd.

Swinscow T. D. V. **Statistics from Square One** 7th edition 1980. BMA Publications Ltd.

THE VIVAS

The Viva Voce examinations for the Part 2 FCAnaesthetists are usually held some weeks after the multiple choice paper. They are currently held at the Royal College of Surgeons, in Lincolns Inn Fields in London, which may entail considerable travelling for many candidates. It is important to arrive at the Viva exam in a cool, mentally collected state of mind, in order to do justice to your knowledge in front of your examiners. The impression you make on the examiners as you arrive at the table cannot help but influence them, so be there in plenty of time, and take a few minutes to recover from the effects of a journey across a large city, before entering the examination hall.

The Examiners
In the part 2 exam the examiners are appointed by the Board of Examiners of the College, from the ranks of consultant anaesthetists, staff of the academic anaesthetic departments, and in some cases, academic pharmacologists and physiologists. This means that you may be examined by an anaesthetist, or by a pharmacologist or physiologist who has never given an anaesthetic. This serves to emphasise the basic scientific nature of this exam. However it remains a part of the exam for an anaesthetic diploma, and as such the physiology and pharmacology relating to anaesthetics figures largely in the questions.

The Format
In the event of your passing the multiple choice paper you will be called for the Viva exams each of which lasts for 20 minutes. You will be given a date and the times of the two vivas. One will be in pharmacology and the other in physiology. The examiners in each subject examine in pairs, one examiner asks questions for approximately ten minutes and then the other examiner takes over for the rest of the time. At the end of the twenty minutes a bell is rung signalling the end of the exam, questions cannot be asked after the bell and answers need not be finished.

The Candidate's Approach
The examiners are going to see a great many candidates in the course of the exam. You need to impress upon them your knowledge of the subject, your ability to apply that knowledge, and your generally professional approach to your work.

Aim to hold their attention and to interest them, look up at the examiners and look interested and keen. Speak audibly and clearly, and if you do not understand the question, say so at once. Do not hesitate for too long, gather your thoughts on the subject and start with the general, commonly known facts; this allows you time to recall the details. Do not jump in with the obscure fact that inevitably leaps into your head, as that route leads to the self dug hole of disaster into which many candidates leap! In the same fashion try to avoid starting with words such as 'possibly' and 'I think'.

Be honest, if you really do not know the answer say so and do not waste time proving your ignorance. No one is capable of knowing everything and you only have twenty minutes to show them what you do know. Do not be put off by being asked a question you cannot answer, take a deep breath and start again on the next question.

If you are asked about a subject that you know well, resist the temptation to tell the examiner all you know and confine yourself to answering the specific question as fully as you can. The examiner will then either draw you further on the subject, in which case you can give as much information as you can, or he will change the subject. Do not despair if the examiner keeps changing the subject, candidates often complain, "I never got going on any subject, they kept changing the topic". This is not necessarily a sign of bad performance, the examiners often do this to candidates in order to test the breadth as well as the depth of their knowledge. Do not forget that the object of the exercise is to answer as many questions correctly as possible, thereby covering a great deal of ground, which enables you to score more points.

In this exam there is a tendency to start off by asking questions about very basic functions at a cellular level, and to go on to the gross or whole body functions, or effects, and finally to the significance in disease or during anaesthesia. Therefore you may well get through a good deal of the exam without discussing the subject of anaesthesia at all, this is quite normal and not a sign that you are failing! Do not despair. Some subjects, statistics, and pharmacokinetics in particular seem to be very unpopular with candidates and very popular with examiners. It is advisable to revise these subjects thoroughly, they are really not that mysterious when studied carefully.

The Preparation

Viva practice is absolutely essential, both in order to improve your technique, and to build up your confidence. Invite your seniors to ask you questions, but try to arrange formal practice vivas. The feeling of sitting down in front of examiners in a separate room and being formally "Viva'd" is quite different from being questioned in the coffee room or

158

during a list. If there are more than one of you preparing for the exam in your hospital it is a very useful and illuminating exercise to watch others having vivas, many faults of technique become obvious when you are not in the 'hot seat'. This type of situation will show you how posture, fidgeting, and long silences can let down even the best prepared candidates.

Finally, the examiners have a difficult job and are always pleased to meet a candidate who is knowledgeable and presents him/herself well. They realise that you are nervous, and really do not set out to trick you. Many examiners think of the answer they want and may continue to question you to obtain that answer; if it seems that you are being asked the same question in several different forms say that you are unclear what he requires rather than waste time. Good preparation and plenty of practice will see you through to the part three.

REVISION INDEX